The Cortisol Connection

Testimonials from SENSE Program Users

(all names have been changed to protect privacy)

"I started SENSE during a *very* stressful time for me—and I expected to gain weight as usual because of the stress.... But SENSE was so simple to follow that it actually made things easier to handle (instead of harder to follow, as is the case with many other diets I have tried).... The program has taught me so much about nutrition and metabolism and how important it is to do several small things at one time to control weight."   — *Sandy*

"My results have been terrific, with a loss of 8 percent body fat and almost twenty pounds. But the best part is that the balance in the plan between exercise and diet and supplements is something I can continue to follow forever."   — *Dennise*

"Dr. Talbott's SENSE program has helped me to lose more than fifty-five pounds of body weight and at least six inches off my waist.... Before starting on SENSE, my stress level was through the roof, I had just bought a bigger belt and I was starting to eye the 46-inch–waist pants (up from my then size 44 and my usual 38).... I can't say enough about how beneficial the program was for me. Aside from the loss of weight and inches, I feel a whole lot better. My mood is up and my stress is way down from where it was at the start of the program."   — *Mitch*

Testimonials (cont'd.)

"By using Dr. Talbott's 'Helping-Hand' approach to eating, I was never hungry, I had *no cravings,* and I never felt like I was on a 'diet' of any kind. By following this program, I have made a complete 180-degree turn with my eating habits—and these changes have benefited my family as well as me."   — *Stephanie*

"I was diagnosed with diabetes a few months before trying SENSE, and my main interest was finding something that would help me control my diabetes. The fact that the program focused partly on controlling blood sugar made it seem like a good thing to try—but I never expected all the wonderful benefits in how I look and feel. By following SENSE, I lost more than five inches off my waist and have gone from a size 22 to a size 16."   — *Laura*

. . . .
.
.
.

Ordering
Trade bookstores in the U.S. and Canada please contact:

Publishers Group West
1700 Fourth Street, Berkeley CA 94710
Phone: (800) 788-3123   Fax: (800) 351-5073

Hunter House books are available at bulk discounts for textbook course adoptions, to qualifying community, health-care, and government organizations, and for special promotions and fund-raising. For details please contact:

Special Sales Department
Hunter House Inc., PO Box 2914, Alameda CA 94501-0914
Phone: (510) 865-5282   Fax: (510) 865-4295
E-mail: ordering@hunterhouse.com

Individuals can order our books from most bookstores,
by calling **(800) 266-5592**, or from our website at
www.hunterhouse.com

The Cortisol Connection

WHY STRESS MAKES YOU FAT
AND RUINS YOUR HEALTH —
AND WHAT YOU CAN DO ABOUT IT

· · · · · · · · · · ·

Shawn Talbott, PH.D.
Foreword by William J. Kraemer, Ph.D.

SECOND EDITION

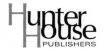

Hunter House PUBLISHERS

Hunter House Inc., Publishers
PO Box 2914
Alameda CA 94501-0914

Library of Congress Cataloging-in-Publication Data
Talbott, Shawn M.
The cortisol connection : why stress makes you fat and ruins your health - and what you can do about it / Shawn Talbott. — 2nd ed.
p. cm.
Includes bibliographical references and index.
ISBN-13: 978-0-89793-492-3 (pbk.)
ISBN-10: 0-89793-492-X (pbk.)
1. Stress management.   2. Stress (Physiology)   3. Hydrocortisone—Physiological effect.   4. Health.   5. Obesity.   I. Title.
RA785.T35 2007
155.9'042—dc22   2007015592

Project Credits

Cover Design	Brian Dittmar Graphic Design
Book Production	John McKercher
Developmental and Copy Editor	Kelley Blewster
Proofreader	John David Marion
Indexer	Nancy D. Peterson
Acquisitions Editor	Jeanne Brondino
Editor	Alexandra Mummery
Senior Marketing Associate	Reina Santana
Rights Coordinator	Candace Groskreutz
Customer Service Manager	Christina Sverdrup
Order Fulfillment	Washul Lakdhon
Administrator	Theresa Nelson
Computer Support	Peter Eichelberger
Publisher	Kiran S. Rana

Printed and Bound by Bang Printing, Brainerd, Minnesota

Manufactured in the United States of America

9 8 7 6 5 4   Second Edition   09 10 11 12 13

Contents

Important Note

The material in this book is intended to provide a review of information regarding the effects of stress and cortisol levels on health. Every effort has been made to provide accurate and dependable information. The contents of this book have been compiled through professional research and in consultation with medical professionals. However, health-care professionals have differing opinions, and advances in medical and scientific research are made very quickly, so some of the information may become outdated.

Therefore, the publisher, authors, and editors, as well as the professionals quoted in the book, cannot be held responsible for any error, omission, or dated material. The authors and publisher assume no responsibility for any outcome of applying the information in this book in a program of self-care or under the care of a licensed practitioner. If you have questions concerning your nutrition or diet, or about the application of the information described in this book, consult a qualified health-care professional.

Foreword

The adrenal hormone cortisol has essentially become how stress is defined. Stress and cortisol have been a topic of intense interest in both the scientific and the lay press for over fifty years. From the pioneering laboratory work of Dr. Hans Selye, a Canadian endocrinologist who first defined stress as a "general adaptation syndrome," to more current views of stress as a specific phenomenon, researchers have always identified cortisol as playing a key role in stress's negative effects. Cortisol plays a wide variety of physiological roles in the body, and when stress produces excessive levels of the hormone, problems result.

In his book *The Cortisol Connection: Why Stress Makes You Fat and Ruins Your Health — and What You Can Do about It*, Dr. Talbott provides important new insights into the physiology of stress, techniques for managing it, and the many innovative methods that can be used to combat stress with nutrition. Dr. Talbott brings scientific credibility to the book by drawing on his extensive experience and understanding of nutrition and stress physiology. The text is well written and easy to understand. It is engaging in its presentation and is an enjoyable read. It is one of the first informative books on this topic suitable for both the lay public and medical professionals.

This book is important to us all because each of us faces a host of stressors in our everyday lives that can potentially increase bodily cortisol levels and affect our health. The importance of nutrition—specifically, the role certain nutritional supplements can play in helping to combat stress and the negative effects of excessive cortisol responses—is one of the hallmarks of Dr. Talbott's work. The book provides valuable information and practical ideas while being carefully crafted to give the reader the understanding and insight necessary to take control of his or her lifestyle to eliminate the negative effects of too much cortisol in the body. I believe this book is a must read for anyone interested in improving his or her health and in coping more effectively with the stresses of life through optimal nutrition.

— William J. Kraemer, Ph.D.
Professor of Kinesiology,
Physiology, and Neurobiology
The University of Connecticut

Acknowledgments

In writing both editions of *The Cortisol Connection*, I have consulted the scientific work of hundreds of researchers and medical professionals, but, in particular, the experiments of the following scientists were especially helpful: Robert Sapolsky, Ph.D., at Stanford University; George Chrousos, M.D., at the National Institutes of Health; Per Bjorntorp, M.D., Ph.D., at the University of Göteborg, in Sweden; Susan Barr, Ph.D., at the University of British Columbia; and Elissa Epel, Ph.D., at the University of California at San Francisco.

The process of writing and revising *The Cortisol Connection* has been a constant project for me over the past five years. My experiences during this period as an educator, textbook author, university professor, and clinic director have helped me to refine and expand my thinking about the impact of stress and cortisol on health. Most of all, I would like to acknowledge that this book would not have been possible without the invaluable participation over the years of the thousands of participants in my SENSE programs. These participants were just like you in many ways: intelligent and curious people who were too busy and too stressed and who were thinking that they needed to do something to get their lives (and bodies) under control. For these folks, *The Cortisol Connection* and the SENSE Lifestyle Program provided the education and the answers they needed to regain the control they were looking for. I owe each of them a huge THANK YOU for helping me to refine my original thinking into the research-proven yet "real-life" program that you will read about in the coming pages.

Finally, I need to thank my most important advocate and supporter—my loving wife and best friend, Julie Talbott. In putting together this book and continually refining the SENSE program, I was often at risk for not following my own advice about controlling my cortisol levels. Despite believing that depriving myself of sleep or drinking too much coffee or skipping a workout might increase my short-term productivity, I also knew quite clearly that these practices would certainly increase my cortisol levels and do "bad things" to me in the long run. Luckily, Julie was always there to provide extra reinforcement and willpower to help me do the right thing and to "follow your own advice!" (her words, including the exclamation point). Julie provides the same balance to my work that she has forever provided to our relationship and to my life—and for that I dedicate this book to her.

Introduction

Back in 2002, when the first edition of this book was published, I started off by asking readers three simple questions:

1. Got stress? Of course you do! That's strike one.

2. How about sleep—do you get at least eight solid hours of restful sleep every night? No? Strike two.

3. What about your diet—are you among the millions of people who are actively dieting or concerned about what you eat? Yes? Strike three.

As you might imagine, most people had three strikes. In our fast-paced, hurry-hurry, twenty-first-century world, almost of all of us are stressed out, sleep deprived, and hyper-concerned about our diet and food choices. Because of this chronic stress, unfortunately, most of us are also fat.

At last count, national health statistics pegged approximately two out of three Americans (65 percent of us) as overweight or obese. People of ideal body weight are a distinct minority (35 percent) in this country.

Health experts have been telling us since the 1950s that the solution to our obesity epidemic is simple: "Eat less and exercise more." But in fifty years of our hearing this party line repeatedly, it has become obvious that this recommendation does not work. People either hear the message and ignore the advice, or they hear the message and they *try* as hard as they can—but fail. In my experience as a nutritional biochemist and weight-loss educator, people *do* hear this message and they really *do* try to eat right and get some exercise. But they fail to lose weight. Why?

The reason for diet failure comes down to one primary cause—stress. Stressed-out people eat more (and eat more junk). Stressed-out people have more belly fat (and thus more diabetes as a result). Stressed-out people exercise less—mostly because they are "time-stressed" and feel they have no time for exercise. Stressed-out people are constantly tired during the day—and yet they can't relax enough to get a good night of sleep. Stressed-out people also have more heart attacks, more depression, more colds, and less sex. I cannot think of a more dismal picture—and stress is at the root of it.

In mid-2005, more than three years after the original edition of this book was written, the *Wall Street Journal* ran an article titled "Stress and Your Waistline" (*Health Journal*, July 19, 2005) that highlighted some of the recent studies showing the link between stress (and cortisol exposure) and abdominal fat accumulation (belly fat). The article explained how controlling stress and cortisol could be beneficial to dieters and could enhance weight-loss results. However, the article concluded by saying that "stress management might be the one weight-loss strategy that society hasn't really addressed." On the contrary, the weight-loss program that my colleagues and I have administered for the last five years employs stress-management and cortisol-control techniques along with diet, exercise, and dietary supplements—and the results for the participants have been nothing short of dramatic.

How is it that something as simple as stress can cause so many problems—from depression to immune suppression to weight gain? The reason is because a chronic stress response, such as the one we mount every day when faced with deadlines, money concerns, traffic, family conflicts, irritating coworkers, and other worries, causes an immediate and profound change in a variety of hormones in our bodies. We used to focus primarily on one stress hormone, cortisol, because it is thought of as the "primary" stress hormone. Now, however, we know that although cortisol is still important to consider, it is clearly only one part of the hormonal and metabolic response to stress and weight gain. Research conducted during the last five years has shown us that cortisol is involved in a complex interplay with another hormone (testosterone) and with a fat-storing enzyme (HSD).

That interplay goes something like this:

1. Stress increases **cortisol** exposure, which in most people leads to increased appetite and abdominal weight gain.

2. Increased cortisol reduces **testosterone** levels in both men and women, leading to a loss of sex drive and muscle mass and an increase in fatigue and body fat.

3. Some people with high stress do not have high levels of cortisol in their blood, but they can still gain weight because of high cortisol levels within fat cells. Fat cells contain an enzyme, called **HSD,** that increases cortisol levels *within* the cell as a way to encourage *more fat storage* (even when cortisol levels in the blood remain normal).

All of this boils down to a very simple strategy for dealing with weight. It may be a bit reminiscent of Bill Clinton's 1992 campaign for president, which is sometimes summarized in a single sound bite: "It's the economy, stupid." If I were to have a sound bite of my own about weight loss, it would be "Stress makes you fat *and* stupid" (because cortisol can also destroy brain cells).

Like many complex problems, the solution is actually not all that complicated—and it looks like this:

1. The "eat less and exercise more" approach to weight loss has failed.

2. Stress makes you fat.

3. Maintain hormonal balance between cortisol (both outside and inside cells) and testosterone.

How can I make such a bold claim—that the solution to the weight-loss puzzle is as simple as three little sound bites? Because for the past five years, hundreds of people in my nutrition clinic and hundreds of thousands of people who have read my books, read my interviews in magazines and newspapers, and seen or heard my appearances on television and radio have realized dramatic benefits with my weight-loss program, dubbed the SENSE program. My SENSE program has been presented at some of the most prestigious scientific research conferences in the world, including the American College of Nutrition, the American Society for Clinical Nutrition, Experimental Biology, the American College of Sports Medicine, and the Obesity Society. It is that exact program that is described in this book.

Our weight-loss breakthrough came after offering the SENSE program to thousands of successful participants for more than 4 years, when we realized that we had been concentrating our efforts too narrowly on controlling cortisol levels in the blood (*outside* of fat cells) and ignoring the fact that cortisol levels *inside* of fat cells might still be too high. By naturally controlling the activity of the fat-storing HSD enzyme within fat cells, we could also control cortisol levels within fat cells and thus remove a potent fat-storage signal. When we combined this inside/outside approach to cortisol control with a natural rebalancing of testosterone levels, magic happened (or at least it appeared that way to our participants). This "magic" was nothing of the sort, but rather was a very precise approach to balancing normal biochemistry and metabolism. Our approach appeared magical to our participants because they felt great, the plan was easy to follow, and it worked. As the scientist and science-fiction writer Arthur C. Clarke so famously stated, "Any sufficiently advanced technology is indistinguishable from magic"—a statement that drives me to constantly advance our biochemical approach to weight loss so I can keep the "magic" happening for people.

Don't get me wrong: Proper diet and regular exercise are still important pieces of the weight-loss puzzle, but they are not the only considerations. We also need to consider the brain (sleep, stress, mood) and hormone levels (cortisol and testosterone) for the most complete approach to truly effective weight loss. How many people try to "eat right" and "exercise more"—and yet still gain weight? Millions! The missing pieces of the puzzle for most people are stress control and hormone control—and adding those pieces has made all the difference in the world for our participants over the years.

With SENSE, you get a proven program that is easy to follow. After five years of tracking results, we have a 91 percent completion rate, while typical weight-loss programs are lucky to achieve 50 percent. Our participants don't just lose weight; they lose significant amounts of body fat, and they feel great doing it because they are learning to control the hormones that have made them hungry, fat, tired, and depressed.

You *have* to feel good to stay on a "diet." If it's a chore, then you quit—simple as that. Our program reduces depression by 52 percent, reduces fatigue by 48 percent, and you feel like a million bucks (overall mood improves by 22 percent). Not only do our participants lose body fat, but they also maintain their muscle mass—so they avoid the common drop in metabolic rate (and subsequent weight gain) seen with other weight-loss programs. This result led one of our participants to remark that the SENSE program wasn't just "metabolic" in its effects, but it was also *mega*-bolic!

Perhaps the biggest problem with chronic stress is the fact that its initial effects are so subtle: Cortisol goes up and testosterone goes down, and before you know it you have a few extra pounds of weight, a slight reduction in energy levels, a modest drop in sex drive, a bit of trouble with memory. Much of the time, we simply brush these effects off as "normal" aspects of aging. However, as *The Cortisol Connection* will show, they are actually the earliest signs of obesity, diabetes, impotence, dementia, heart disease, cancer, and many related conditions. Indeed, stress is emerging as a key factor in the very process we all recognize as "aging."

Bad news, to be sure, but the good news is that you can do something about it, and this is where *The Cortisol Connection* can help. Through the easy-to-follow SENSE program you learn how to incorporate stress management, exercise, nutrition, and dietary supplements into a realistic (that is, very doable) approach to controlling stress and maintaining cortisol and testosterone levels. (Our most recent study showed a 15 percent improvement in bodily levels of these hormones.)

I feel very strongly—in fact, I am *certain*—that once you understand the relationship between modern stressors, your cortisol/ testosterone levels, and their effects on your long-term health, you will be motivated to do something about getting your metabolism back into balance.

But first, let's see if you qualify for the program: Let's check your exposure to stress and your risk for developing what I call a "Type C" personality (C for cortisol). The Type C personality, a term I coined during the writing of the first edition of *The Cortisol Connection,* is characterized by always feeling rushed, busy, and chronically stressed.

ARE YOU A TYPE C?
GAUGING YOUR EXPOSURE TO STRESS

Unless you are fully attuned to listening to your body, as an elite athlete may be accustomed to doing, it can be very difficult to read the telltale signs associated with stress-induced health problems, such as those described in the preceding few paragraphs. Therefore, it may be helpful to gauge your overall exposure to stress using the simple questionnaire presented below, which I call the Type C Self-Test. We have used this questionnaire for the past five years to measure stress levels and the stress-controlling effects of the SENSE program. This series of questions can help you decide whether your body may be exposed to excessive stress and cortisol levels on a regular basis.

Type C Self-Test

Directions:

- For each question, write your score in the corresponding column.
- For each answer of Never/No, give yourself zero (0) points.
- For each answer of Occasionally, give yourself one (1) point.
- For each answer of Frequently/Yes, give yourself two (2) points.
- Add all the numbers in each column.
- Add each of the three column's totals together for your total score.
- Your total score indicates your Type C Index.

Question   Never *or* No (0 points) / Occasionally (1 point) / Frequently *or* Yes (2 points)

How often do you experience stressful situations?   _____

How often do you feel tired or fatigued for no apparent reason?   _____

How often do you get **less than** eight hours of sleep?   _____

How often do you feel anxious/depressed?   _____

How often do you feel overwhelmed or confused?   _____

How often is your sex drive lower than you would like it to be?   _____

Do you tend to gain weight easily?   _____

Are you currently dieting?   _____

How often have you attempted to control your body weight?   _____

How often do you pay close attention to the foods you eat?   _____

How often do you crave carbohydrates (sweets and/or breads)?   _____

How often do you experience difficulty with memory or concentration?   _____

How often do you experience tension headaches or muscle tightness
in your neck, shoulders, or jaw?   _____

How often do you experience digestive problems such as gas,
bloating, ulcers, heartburn, constipation, or diarrhea?   _____

How often do you get sick/catch colds or the flu?   _____

SCORE (add all numbers together)   _____ *points*

Cortisol Index

Total Score	Type C Index	Comments
0–5 points	**Relaxed Jack** (Low risk, no worries)	You are cool as a cucumber and have either a very low level of stress or a tremendous ability to deal effectively with incoming stressors. Keep doing whatever you're doing!
6–10 points	**Strained Jane** (Moderate risk)	You *may be* suffering from an overactive stress response and chronically elevated levels of cortisol and should incorporate antistress strategies into your lifestyle whenever possible—but don't stress out about it!
Greater than 10 points	**Stressed Jess** (High risk)	You are *almost definitely* suffering from an overactive stress response, chronically elevated levels of cortisol, and its detrimental metabolic effects—and you need to take immediate steps to regain control.

Are you a Stressed Jess? These days, who isn't? Consider the fact that virtually anybody who experiences stress on a regular basis, gets less than eight hours of sleep each night, or is either dieting or concerned about what they eat is on the fast track to elevated cortisol levels.

This is not to say that the Stressed Jesses among us are going to keel over tomorrow from cortisol overexposure—nor does it mean that the rare Relaxed Jacks will necessarily live to a ripe old age. What it does mean is that each of us can benefit from targeted cortisol control. Sometimes your cortisol-control regimen needs to be more aggressive (such as during times of particularly high stress), while at other times you'll have less stress in your life and you can let your attention to cortisol control wander a bit (such as during your vacation to Tahiti).

The bottom line is that living in the twenty-first century brings along with it a certain amount of unavoidable stress—and with that stress comes elevated cortisol levels and depressed testosterone levels. It is how we deal with that stress and what we do to control those hormone levels that make the difference when it comes to our long-term health. So keep reading. Whatever your score on the Type C Self-Test, *The Cortisol Connection: Why Stress Makes You Fat and Ruins Your Health — and What You Can Do about It* was written for you.

CHAPTER 1

Stress and Your Health: The Type C Personality

Perhaps one of the most poignant realizations in health and medical research during the last two or three decades is that our bodies, including our nervous systems and endocrine (hormonal) systems, were simply not meant for the unique stresses that we face as part of our everyday life in the twenty-first century. The series of daily events that I refer to as the "twenty-first-century syndrome" leads most of us to experience a state of perpetual stress—that familiar feeling of always being "on" and rushed and harried and frantic. In other words, that stressed-out feeling that you have every day may be "typical" because everyone else is experiencing it, but it is *not* "normal" in a physiological sense, nor is it associated with good health.

In the Introduction I presented the term "Type C personality" and defined such an individual as someone who is chronically stressed and, thus, chronically exposed to elevated levels of the stress hormone cortisol (the C in "Type C" stands for "cortisol"). Here are some characteristics of the Type C personality (a.k.a. the twenty-first-century syndrome). Which of them can you identify with?

- In a perpetual state of "hurry hurry"

- Twenty-five hours of stuff to do in a twenty-four-hour day
- Low-grade cortisol overexposure
- Depression
- Fatigue
- Low sex drive
- Trouble concentrating
- Abdominal weight gain

As dismal as these characteristics sound, the good news is that we have a broad array of tools at our disposal for both combating stress and reducing the detrimental effects of stress hormones on our bodies—and that is what this book is all about.

Consider for a moment that the incidence of depression and anxiety in our society is now ten times higher than it was just a generation ago. Is this staggering increase due to physicians diagnosing these "diseases" at a higher rate because now they have drugs to "cure" them? Or is it due to the fact that many of us are simply living lives that feel out of our control? This same state of being overly stressed has resulted in close to ninety million cases of diseases with "no known cause," such as chronic fatigue syndrome, fibromyalgia, irritable bowel syndrome (IBS), recurrent yeast infections, autoimmune disease, chronic back pain, and other "nonspecific" conditions. In each of these cases, the *obvious* cause is the unrelenting stress under which we toil on a daily basis, yet Western medicine is often slow to admit that "mental" conditions such as stress can have physical effects upon the rest of the body. Nonetheless, even though our modern medical establishment has been excruciatingly slow in appreciating the very real impact of stress on overall health and wellness, the worldwide research community has made remarkable strides during the last thirty years in uncovering deeper and more direct links between stress and disease. So strong are these links, in fact, that an entirely new branch of science has developed that is called *psychoneuroendocrinology*, a term that denotes the close link between the mind ("psycho-," what we think), the nervous system ("neuro-," how those thoughts are transmitted as nerve impulses throughout the body), and the hormonal system ("endocrin-," which controls functions and behaviors in all areas of the body).

How do I know that stress is an epidemic in this country? One reason is because each of the top ten drugs prescribed in the United States is for a stress-related disease, for example depression, anxiety, insomnia, diabetes, heartburn, high blood pressure, and immune-system suppression (antibiotics).

Most readers will understand on some level that too much stress is "bad"; after all, our grandmothers knew that. But those same readers might be surprised to learn that you don't have to "change your life" as advocated by so many of the "self-help" set. Don't get me wrong here: Reducing your exposure to stress is never anything but good—but it is also important to understand that you can live a completely frantic, out-of-control, stress-filled life (as I do) and enjoy (almost) every minute of it (as I do) while also enhancing your health and performance through the kind of targeted stress management, exercise, nutrition, and supplementation that you will read about throughout this book (as I do).

ARE YOU HAPPY?

Are you happier now than you were last year? Five years ago? If you're like most people, your level of happiness has declined significantly, while your "anxiety index" (things you worry about) has increased (also significantly). Across the American population, the number of people who identify themselves as "very happy" with their lives has declined by about 60 percent within the last fifty years. Why were people in the 1950s happier? Less stress, fewer hours of work, and a higher comparative standard of living. In the past twenty-five years, the average American workweek has blossomed to fifty hours from forty hours, a level higher than any European country and equal to that of Japan. Even with those extra hours of work, we are *behind* in our ability to maintain the same overall standard of living of twenty-five years ago (or at least it feels that way when we take into consideration the fact that most of us want to improve our lives and the lives of our kids). Talk about stress! We're all working longer and harder than our parents did—and yet we're not able to live up to the same (comparative) standard of living we had as kids. Those ten extra hours of work have gained us nothing in terms of security or living standards.

We're spinning our wheels, and yet even more seems to be expected of us. We need to be the best worker, the best mom, drive the best car, live in the best neighborhood and the best house, eat at the best restaurants—and it is driving many of us to an early burnout. We even see it in our kids, who go from school or day care to the babysitter to soccer to homework at the same frantic pace. Is there any mystery behind the rise in Ritalin and Prozac use in American kids or the rise in the diagnosis of ADHD (attention deficit hyperactivity disorder)?

In a survey conducted in 2006 by the New York Academy of Medicine and the National Association of Social Workers, only about 20 percent of women between the ages of thirty-five and fifty-four rated themselves as "very happy," a lower proportion than that found in other groups of Americans. Money, time, and health concerns loomed large in the survey. Fifty-five percent indicated that they had "difficulty managing stress" in their personal lives.

Perhaps one of the most potent and prevalent stressors in our modern society is money. Researchers refer to a "worry about money" as "socioeconomic stress" (SES), and dozens upon dozens of new studies are showing us that SES is associated not only with elevated cortisol levels but also with increased risk for heart disease, weight gain, and diabetes. In one study conducted by researchers at Carnegie Mellon University, in Pittsburgh, individuals with higher levels of "money stress" had higher cortisol levels. (They also smoked more and skipped breakfast more often.) Scientists at Brandeis University, in Boston, have shown that the highest cortisol levels are found in older adults suffering from money stress.

Ask any of your friends about the things that stress them out the most, and the issue of money is sure to come up. Making it, spending it, balancing bills, etc.—money is undoubtedly one of the primary sources of stress for all of us. Researchers from the University College of London, in England, have assessed the impact of changes in financial strain. They looked at people who made more or less money than one year prior and found that individuals with "improved" (less) financial strain also had lower cortisol and reduced blood pressure.

I know that it would be very politically correct of me to tell you that you need to "dial it back a notch"—to stop and smell the roses, decompress, work fewer hours, take on less debt, and all the rest. But I won't. Instead, I will acknowledge that each of these approaches affords some very real benefits, but I will also acknowledge that "dialing it back a notch" is completely impractical for most people. I can certainly tell you how great the various approaches to "destressing" your life may be, but I know that you'll most likely roll your eyes and go on with your high-stress, hurry-hurry, frantic pace—and I will not have helped you at all.

Rather than focusing most of my efforts on preaching to you about something that I know you'll probably ignore, I will instead focus the bulk of my recommendations on some proven approaches to using minimal exercise, simple nutrition, and natural dietary supplements to control the biochemistry underlying your stress response. I will also offer up a few simple stress-management techniques that you can implement without drastically changing your lifestyle. By following some of my suggestions, you can reduce the detrimental effects of stress on your metabolism—meaning you can lose weight, boost your energy levels, enhance your mood, and improve your sex life—without having to sacrifice your current lifestyle (or become a monk).

THE "NORMAL" STRESS RESPONSE

There you are, a zebra strolling across the African savanna. You're minding your own business, maybe looking for some tender young grasses to satisfy your appetite, when suddenly A LION COMES CHARGING TOWARD YOU FROM THE BUSHES! This is the classic scenario used to describe the stress response, otherwise known as the "fight-or-flight" response. In reaction to the charging lion, your body quickly paces itself through a series of neurological, biochemical, hormonal, and physiological actions, each of which is designed to help you run away from that lion and survive for another day.

In the case of the zebra, the stress response runs its complete course, from start to finish, in a relatively short period of time (see Figure 1.1). The stress occurs (the charging lion), which causes the zebra's brain and hormone system to release a series of stress hormones (the stress response), which enables it to fight off the lion or

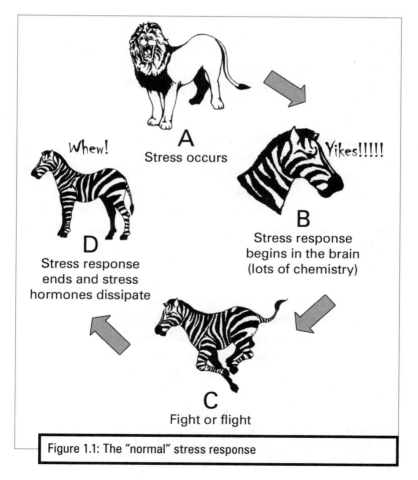

Figure 1.1: The "normal" stress response

run away from it (the fight-or-flight response). After getting away from the lion, the zebra's stress hormones return to normal—end of story.

Unfortunately, we humans aren't so lucky. The vast majority of our daily stressors come from things that are much scarier than vicious lions—things like monthly mortgage payments, credit card bills, project deadlines, traffic jams, family commitments—the list goes on. The major problem with our modern-day stressors is that they are less easy to escape from than the charging lion. The things that cause us stress today are difficult to fight off and impossible to run away from—and they also seem to keep coming back again and again. This unfortunate situation puts us in the position of being stuck midway through the normal stress response, where stress hormones are chronically elevated (see Figure 1.2).

In this scenario, our modern, fast-paced, high-stress lifestyles cause us to become stuck between steps B and C, creating what can be referred to as the "Type C" personality: a victim of chronic stress and elevated cortisol. You have probably heard of the "Type A" and "Type B" personalities. Type A's are stereotyped as high-strung stress monsters, and Type B's are cast as laid-back folks who always roll with the punches. It may be obvious to you that nobody is either a "pure" Type A or Type B personality; rather, we are all a blend of the two, some with a bit more "A" and others with a bit more "B" thrown in.

Unfortunately, we are *all* vulnerable to chronic stress and can become a Type C personality if we aren't careful to control either our *exposure* to stress or the way in which our bodies *respond* to stress. The "C" in the Type C designation also refers to the name of the primary stress hormone—cortisol—which is elevated during periods of high stress. When we encounter something (anything) that causes us to feel stress, our cortisol levels go up. If we experience stressful events on a regular basis and are unable to effectively rid ourselves of the stressor, our cortisol levels stay constantly elevated above normal levels.

Yes, you may say, bills, traffic, and the demands of work and family are all things that cause us to worry and to feel stress, but

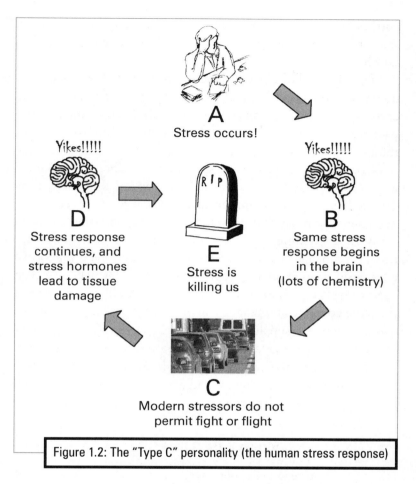

Figure 1.2: The "Type C" personality (the human stress response)

they're not exactly as life-threatening as a hungry lion bearing down on you—or are they? In cases of *acute* stress—someone sneaking up behind you and shouting "BOO!"—there are probably no long-term health consequences. In cases of *chronic* stress, however, when you ruminate, obsess, and continually mull over the "what if's" of a stressful situation, you put yourself into the Type C condition of having chronically elevated cortisol levels.

Over the long term, elevated cortisol levels can be as detrimental to overall health as elevated cholesterol is for heart disease or excessive blood sugar is for diabetes. Aside from that, elevated cortisol levels make you fat, kill your sex drive, shrink your brain, squelch your immune system, and generally make you feel terrible. So what to do?

Luckily, you have lots of choices. The easiest choice of all is to do nothing (like most people) and let chronic stress and elevated cortisol levels slowly break down your bodily defenses and increase your risk for disease. The more difficult choices are to do something—about either your stress level, the way you handle stress, or how your body responds to stressful situations. There have been at least a gazillion self-help books and empowering seminars on the general topic of "stress management," so you'll get very little of that here. Suffice it to say that stress is a "bad thing" and stress management is a "good thing"—but because of the complexities of the topics of psychological and emotional coping, developing supportive relationships, and honoring your inner self (all of which have been dealt with effectively in other books), this book will stick to some of the more concrete and practical approaches to dealing with stress: diet, exercise, and supplements.

Before we get too far into a discussion of what you can do to get a handle on your chronic stress and elevated cortisol levels, let's talk briefly about what stress is and how it relates to your cortisol levels and overall health profile.

WHAT IS STRESS?

It's not as if you've never experienced stress. Each of us encounters stress in one form or another on a daily basis—in fact, we encounter stress multiple times during every day of our lives. Even more important than the *things* that cause us to experience stress, however, is our body's ability to *cope* with that stress. We're going to talk about the physiological and biochemical responses of your body to the things we identify as "stress" and about how you can customize your approach to dealing with those internal chemical cascades.

Let's start off with a tidy definition of stress. For our purposes we'll define it as "what you feel when life's demands exceed your ability to meet those demands." With that said, it is important to acknowledge that everybody has a different capacity to effectively cope with stress and, thus, to "perform" when stress is encountered. Even those rare individuals who have a high tolerance for accommodating stressful situations ultimately have a breaking point. Add enough total stress to *anybody* and performance suffers.

Many of the top stress researchers in the world have made the interesting distinction between the type of stressors faced by our cousins in the animal kingdom (short-term or *acute* stressors) and the kind we modern humans routinely face (longer-term and repeated *chronic* stressors). To compound our problems as "higher" animals, we are plagued not only by physical stressors but also by psychological and social stressors. Some of those psychological stressors are quite real (like your monthly rent or mortgage payment), while others are purely imaginary (like the stressful encounters that you *imagine* you might have with your boss, coworkers, kids, or others). How do you like that? Not only has our large, complex, and supposedly "advanced" brain developed the capacity to get us *out* of a whole lot of stressful situations, but it has also developed the capacity to actually *create* stressful situations where none existed before.

Robert Sapolsky, author of perhaps the best (and most readable) book on the subject of stress physiology, *Why Zebras Don't Get Ulcers* (see Resources, located in the back of the book), uses the whimsical examples of zebras being stressed out by lions and baboons being stressed out by each other to illustrate the fact that short-term (acute) periods of stress are vital to survival (at least from the zebra's perspective). From his many examples, we come to learn that whereas acute periods of stress are necessary, a chronically elevated stress response is detrimental to long-term health in a variety of ways. Following the lead of Dr. Sapolsky and virtually every physiology professor who teaches about the fight-or-flight response, this book will also employ numerous examples of zebras, monkeys, and baboons to illustrate concepts related to stress physiology.

HUMANS ARE NOT ZEBRAS

Here's a vitally important point that we will come back to again and again: Human beings were simply *not* meant to carry around constant disturbances in our stress response (chronic stress); we were built to respond to stress quickly and then to have the stress hormones dissipate immediately (acute stress). When our bodies are exposed to wave after wave of stress (from our modern lifestyles), they begin to break down.

Animals don't normally harbor chronic stress the way humans do, but when they do (during stress experiments, starvation, injury, etc.) they get sick just like humans. In study after study, it quickly becomes obvious that the stress response, while acting as our friend in certain situations, turns against us when "everyday" events are perceived by the body as "stressful" events. Over time, stress-related diseases result from either an overexaggerated stress response (too much response to what should have been a small stressor) or an underexaggerated ability to shut down the stress response (which causes cortisol levels to remain elevated for longer than they should).

STRESS, CORTISOL, AND METABOLISM

This is probably as good a place as any to introduce the concept that cortisol is not a purely toxic substance—although in most cases too much of it certainly wreaks bodily havoc. In many ways, cortisol can be thought of as functioning like cholesterol or insulin: A small amount of each of these substances is needed for the proper functioning of the body. Cholesterol is needed for steroid metabolism. Insulin is necessary for blood-sugar control. And cortisol is needed for the restoration of energy stores following stress. However, if levels of any of these vital compounds exceed a certain small amount for a significant period of time, you run into problems (blocked arteries in the case of high cholesterol, diabetes in the case of elevated insulin, and obesity and a host of chronic diseases in the case of cortisol).

The whole point here is balance—keeping cortisol levels from falling too low or rising too high. In a condition called Addison's disease, people are unable to secrete glucocorticoids (of which cortisol is one) from the adrenal glands. As a result of this inability to mount an effective stress response, people with Addison's disease basically go into a state of shock when faced with a stressful event. They sustain a drop in blood pressure, circulatory collapse, and other such symptoms. So just as you do not want cortisol levels to rise too high, neither do you want them to drop too low.

Whenever you're exposed to stress, be it physical stress, such as exercise or emotional stress (e.g., the kind caused by that guy cutting you off in rush-hour traffic), your body begins a complex cascade of events that can alter metabolism in a number of significant ways. Think again about the fight-or-flight mechanism, wherein stimulatory hormones are secreted to prepare the body for rapid action against (fight) or away from (flight) a particular stressor. In a similar manner, upon exposure to everyday stressors the human body ramps up production of cortisol through a complicated series of events that involves both the hypothalamus and the pituitary glands in the brain (more on that later).

One of cortisol's many functions is to stimulate the release of glucose, fats, and amino acids for energy production. In the liver, cortisol stimulates the breakdown of glycogen into glucose. In the adipose tissue (where we store body fat), fatty acids are released in response to cortisol stimulation. (Fat breakdown? Sounds good, but the longer-term effect is fat gain.) In the skeletal muscles, cortisol promotes the release of amino acids, which are either used directly by the muscle for energy or sent to the liver for conversion into glucose. The main problem with this last scenario, however, is that if it continues for any prolonged period of time, a significant amount of muscle mass may be lost (bad for long-term weight maintenance).

STRESS AND DISEASE

Scientific research and medical evidence clearly show that a sustained high level of cortisol, triggered by chronic unrelenting stress, has debilitating effects on long-term health. Among these many effects is an increase in appetite and cravings for certain foods. Because one of the primary roles of cortisol is to encourage the body to refuel itself after responding to a stressor, an elevated cortisol level keeps your appetite ramped up—so you feel hungry almost all the time. In addition, the type of fat that accumulates as a result of this stress-induced appetite will typically locate itself in the abdominal region of the body (probably so it is readily available for the next stress response). The major problem with abdominal fat, aside from the fact that nobody wants a potbelly, is that this type of fat is also highly associated with the development of heart disease, diabetes, and cancer.

Elevated cortisol levels resulting from chronic stress have been associated with the following conditions:
- Increased appetite and food cravings
- Increased body fat
- Decreased muscle mass
- Decreased bone density
- Increased anxiety
- Increased depression
- Mood swings (anger and irritability)
- Reduced libido (sex drive)
- An impaired immune response
- Memory and learning impairment
- Increased symptoms of PMS—premenstrual syndrome (cramps, increased appetite)
- Increased menopausal side effects (hot flashes, night sweats)

Researchers from around the world have slowly been uncovering the relationship between elevated cortisol levels and numerous chronic health ailments (listed in the sidebar, above). Because of the complex relationships between lifestyle, psychology, and physiology, it is not always possible to determine whether elevated cortisol levels are the primary cause of the chronic health ailment or a mediating factor in the body's response to the chronic health ailment. For example, a powerful synthetic form of cortisol, called cortisone, is used as a drug to reduce swelling, inflammation, and joint pain in cases of rheumatoid arthritis (and it performs these actions quite effectively). The catch here is that cortisone use is typically limited to a short period of time, because long-term exposure leads to memory problems, weight gain, depression, and increased infections, making some people feel that they'd be better off with the painful, swollen joints instead of the long-term side effects of the drug.

CORTISOL: TOO MUCH OR TOO LITTLE?

As mentioned above, just as *over*exposure to cortisol is detrimental to health, so is *under*exposure. Consider the effect of cortisol on the brain. We've known about the links between stress and depression for decades. In the United States alone, stress-related depression accounts for more than thirty billion dollars in medical expenses and lost productivity annually. Researchers at the Institute of Psychiatry at King's College, in London, have determined that stress-related depression actually progresses in two distinct phases. The first phase is characterized by an *overexposure* to cortisol, creating a "toxic" effect whereby too much cortisol actually destroys crucial brain cells responsible for good mood. The second phase is a compensatory mechanism where the brain becomes *resistant* to the effects of cortisol as a way to "protect" itself from cortisol's damaging effects. So the brain cells (neurons) are deprived of cortisol, creating a dramatic *underexposure* that leads to a host of memory and psychological problems. Unfortunately, this syndrome of cortisol resistance leads to a deepening of depression and symptoms of fatigue and confusion, a combination that is very much like the symptoms seen in people with PTSD (posttraumatic stress disorder).

In many ways, you can think of the good/bad aspects of cortisol exposure as you might think of the good/bad aspects of getting too little, enough, or too much exercise. Some is good, but too little or too much are bad. Exercise increases cortisol levels, but this short-term increase in cortisol (similar to the effects of short-term, acute stress) is *good* for immune function, memory, appetite control, weight loss, sexual health, energy levels, inflammation levels, etc. A total lack of exercise makes you fat and dumb (similar to too much cortisol), and too much exercise is like PTSD (cortisol underexposure) because you get hurt easily and your body cannot respond adequately. Greek researchers have shown us that well-trained athletes have high cortisol during their workouts, but that those levels fall back to normal during rest. Overtrained athletes (who are overstressed), on the other hand, have low levels of cortisol during exercise, but high levels during rest, indicating that their bodies are still under stress, perhaps from injury or infection or inadequate recovery from/adaptation to training. They also experience fatigue, weight gain, depressed mood, and poor physical and mental performance.

Because of the close link between stress and depression, every major pharmaceutical company in the world is attempting to develop new drugs to modulate or balance cortisol exposure. The current antidepressant drugs work primarily on serotonin levels in the brain, and some newer ones also increase norepinephrine levels— but none of them address cortisol exposure. This means that only about one-half of the people who try antidepressant drugs obtain any relief from their depression (yet these drugs *still* accounted for almost thirteen billion dollars in sales last year). Among the drug companies that are furiously trying to come up with a pharmaceutical answer for stressed-out people with disrupted cortisol balance are Bristol-Myers Squibb, GlaxoSmithKline, Pfizer, Sanofi-Aventis, Johnson and Johnson, Merck, and Novartis. Several of these companies already make an antidepressant drug that increases serotonin levels, including Pfizer (Zoloft), Eli Lilly (Prozac and Cymbalta), Glaxo (Paxil), and Wyeth (Effexor). But because these drugs are only effective about one half of the time, and because they now have to carry a "black box" warning due to their extreme side effects, including an increased risk of suicide, the pharmaceutical industry needs a new cash cow—and cortisol control looks like the next target.

COUNTERACTING THE EFFECTS
OF CHRONIC STRESS

So who has elevated cortisol levels? Lots of people. But to narrow it down, the Type C Self-Test included in the Introduction provides a convenient and fairly reliable gauge of a person's exposure to stress and, consequently, of his or her risk for elevated cortisol levels. We have used this very same Type C Self-Test in a number of research studies in my Utah nutrition clinic, and the results we've seen track almost identically with results from more extensive psychological surveys as well as with measures of salivary cortisol.

So take the Type C Self-Test to determine whether you're a Strained Jane, a Stressed Jess, or a Relaxed Jack. Discovering this basic information is a first step in figuring out what you can do to counteract the effects of chronic stress. As mentioned earlier in the chapter, there are numerous approaches for doing so.

For example, many forms of stress management exist, and there are many fine references available on that topic (see the Resources section at the back of the book for a selected listing). This book takes the view that although stress-management techniques have been around for decades, very few of these regimens have made a large impact on the health or well-being of the average person. Why is this true? Are the techniques ineffective? No, many of them work perfectly well—*if* you can put them into practice. For the vast majority of people, however, wedging another stress-management tool into their already busy lives does little more than add further stress. I know that some stress-management gurus will disagree with me, but from a purely practical point of view (from my position as a nutritional biochemist and an educator), most people can't be bothered with traditional approaches to stress management. Many of us can't even be bothered to exercise or eat the way we know we should—both of which could go a long way toward reducing the detrimental effects of stress on our bodies.

So what else can we do? Lots! Reading *The Cortisol Connection* is a good start. First we lay the foundation: Chapters 2 through 6 flesh out the relationship between modern lifestyles, stress, cortisol (the primary stress hormone), HSD (a fat-storing enzyme), testosterone (an "antistress" hormone), and a wide range of health problems. Next, the book focuses on presenting ways to counteract stress and the damaging effects of cortisol. The focus begins in Chapter 7 with an introduction to the SENSE Lifestyle Program. SENSE stands for the five key methods for dealing with stress: **S**tress management, **E**xercise, **N**utrition, **S**upplementation, and **E**valuation.

A prominent focus of this book is upon the use of natural dietary supplements. Specifically, Chapter 8 outlines the supplements that are known to effectively and safely influence the stress response—from general relaxation to specific modulation of the hormones and enzymes involved in cortisol metabolism. Each supplement is described in terms of the scientific and medical evidence for its effects on increasing or decreasing cortisol exposure. Recommendations for safety, dosage levels, and what to look for if you decide to use the supplement are also provided. This information-rich chapter can be thought of as sort of a handbook of supplements for cortisol control. Some readers will prefer to use it as a reference they can consult as needed, while others will read it straight through to gain as much knowledge as possible about the different options they have for controlling cortisol.

Chapter 9 brings all of the information together in a detailed discussion of the SENSE Lifestyle Program. There you will read about real people who have used various aspects of SENSE to literally transform their lives (making "sense" out of them, so to speak).

The Cortisol Connection includes several case studies of individuals who have experienced benefits from using diet, exercise, and nutritional supplements to control their cortisol levels. Perhaps you will relate to one or more of them as experiencing some of the same stressors and life situations as you do—and perhaps some aspects of their approach to cortisol control will help you come up with your own cortisol-control plan.

WHY SUPPLEMENTS?

Why *not* supplements? A strategic regimen of carefully chosen natural dietary supplements can help control stress, reduce cortisol levels, provide relaxation and more restful sleep, help balance blood sugar, promote weight loss, and boost the immune system. For most of us, from a purely practical perspective, following a balanced cortisol-control regimen that incorporates appropriate dietary supplementation is a lot more "doable" than a complicated stress-management program or a time-consuming exercise regimen. Again, this does not at all imply that stress management is unimportant or that supplements can provide all of the same benefits delivered by exercise. It simply means that supplements, for the majority of people, represent something they can realistically incorporate into their already busy daily lives and that can have a powerfully beneficial impact on controlling stress and balancing cortisol levels.

Many of the dietary supplements covered in this book have been used for centuries as part of traditional medicinal regimens. In some cases the modern scientific evidence for a beneficial health effect of a supplement is quite strong, while in other cases the evidence is weak or nonexistent. Chapter 8 will guide you through the supplements that appear to hold the most promise in terms of controlling the stress response and counteracting some of the detrimental effects of chronically elevated cortisol.

SUMMARY

After reading this chapter, you are probably more than a little concerned about your future health. However, instead of letting concern grow into worry and worry grow into stress, you can do something about your situation. Maybe you just need to eat better. Or maybe you could benefit from taking a balanced multivitamin tablet. Perhaps you could use a specific cortisol-controlling supplement—or even an entire program designed to control your stress and cortisol levels. Whatever your individual cortisol-control needs happen to be, the information in this book will help you address them. Your first step toward improved health and lifelong wellness starts on the next page. Good luck!

CHAPTER 2

The Science of Stress

B ecause our modern world rarely requires the evolutionary
fight-or-flight response to stress, we deny our bodies their
natural physical reaction to stress. Unfortunately, the brain
still registers stress in the same way as it always has, but because we
no longer react to that stress with vigorous physical activity (fighting or running away), our bodies store the stress response and continue to churn out high levels of stress hormones. Before we know
it, we're living the "Type C" lifestyle, characterized by chronic stress
and consistently elevated cortisol levels.

In one of the more ironic twists visited upon us humans as
"higher" animals, our brains are so "well developed" that our bodies have learned to respond to *psychological* stress with the same
hormonal cascade that happens with exposure to a *physical* stressor. This means that just by our thinking about a stressful event,
even if that event is highly unlikely to actually occur, our endocrine
system gets all in an uproar. Bad news to be sure, but the upside to
this story is that even though psychological variables can trigger
the stress response, good evidence exists that we can also harness
the mind to *counteract* some aspects of the stress response by using
biofeedback and similar relaxation techniques.

Many stress physiologists believe that it is our degree of cortisol *variability* that indicates a healthy stress response: neither high

cortisol nor low cortisol, but a cortisol level that fluctuates normally in response to stress and relaxation. Chronically high cortisol is bad and chronically low cortisol is also bad—but "flat" levels seem to be just as bad as either extreme. A cortisol rhythm that is responsive and variable is good—meaning low at night and low when relaxed, but high during acute stress, and high during exercise, and high during a work deadline, but recovering to baseline levels quickly. We *do not* want cortisol to be chronically anything (high or low or medium), but rather, we want cortisol *flux*. We want a highly responsive, finely tuned pattern of cortisol activity.

In the last few years, stress research has shifted away from simply measuring whether cortisol levels are "high" or "low" to focus on how those levels fluctuate over time. In many cases of stress overload, a pattern of "flat" cortisol rhythm is observed. This means that cortisol levels are within ranges that we might call "normal," but they do not appear to go up in response to stress, or to fall when we're supposed to be relaxed. The result is that our bodies are constantly exposed to moderate levels of cortisol on a twenty-four-hour basis, a situation that we are learning may be the worst-case scenario for long-term health. For example, people with chronic stress diseases such as chronic fatigue syndrome and fibromyalgia are known to exhibit a "flat" cortisol rhythm, as are sufferers of PTSD and children who have suffered physical abuse. Additionally, German researchers have found that when cortisol rhythms become flattened, the HSD (fat-storing) system (discussed in Chapter 4) kicks into overdrive, so that abdominal fat cells still "see" a high cortisol level (and thus store fat even faster), while the rest of the body "sees" normal ranges of cortisol (albeit at a constant and never fluctuating level).

STRESSED VERSUS STRESSED OUT: WHAT'S THE DIFFERENCE?

The difference between being "stressed" and being "stressed out" is that being stressed induces an adaptive response (cortisol goes up and then comes down), whereas being stressed out suggests an inability to mount a normal stress response (cortisol rhythm stays flat, so overall cortisol exposure over twenty-four hours is actually higher). It is this nonadaptive cortisol response that scientists at Rockefeller University, in New York, believe leads to most of the common diseases of modern life. Dutch neurology researchers have also observed the same pattern of flattened cortisol rhythm and nonadaptive stress response in chronic fatigue, fibromyalgia, PTSD, depression, and burnout.

The Type C personality, a term that I coined in the first edition of *The Cortisol Connection,* has also been called the Type D personality (D for "distressed") by researchers from Columbia University. Like my "always rushed and always busy" Type C person, Columbia's Type D is "characterized by the joint tendency to experience negative emotions and to inhibit these emotions while avoiding social contacts with others." This means Type D people have more of a "depressed" personality than the harried Type C's. The similarity between C's and D's, however, is their overexposure to cortisol, leading some people to feel constantly busy and others to feel depressed. Indeed, researchers from the University of Pennsylvania have recently shown a strong and direct link between stress and tissue breakdown in the brain and in skeletal structures. The Penn scientists found a dramatic association between high cortisol, depression, and reduced bone density—with up to 67 percent of the association between depression and bone density being attributed to stress-induced changes in cortisol levels.

STAGES OF STRESS

When the brain perceives a stressful event, it responds by stimulating endocrine glands throughout the body to release hormones, including both adrenaline and cortisol. Adrenaline is responsible for the "up" feeling that causes excitement, while cortisol is responsible for modulating the way our bodies use various fuel sources. Cortisol is known as a *glucocorticoid* because it is secreted by the adrenal cortex (thus *corticoid*) and because it increases levels of blood sugar, or glucose (thus *gluco*corticoid).

The work of the "father" of stress research, scientist Hans Selye, provides some of the earliest evidence of what we now know as the classic model for adaptation to stress. During experimentation with rats, he observed that given *any* source of external biological stress, an organism would respond with a predictable biological pattern in an attempt to restore its internal homeostasis. In other words, if stress knocks us out of balance, then our bodies will go through a series of steps (the stress response) to help us regain that balance. He termed this struggle to maintain balance the "general adaptation syndrome," and although modern researchers do not agree with every detail of Selye's stress paradigm, his original division of the stress response into three categories is useful for our purposes in understanding what we can do to combat stress.

Selye proposed that the general adaptation syndrome was the body's way of reacting to a stressor to bring the body's systems back into balance. The first phase of the response, which is termed the *alarm* phase, is characterized by an immediate activation of the nervous system and adrenal glands; this is the sudden "jolt" that a stressor delivers to the body. Next comes a phase of *resistance*, which is characterized by activation of the hypothalamic-pituitary-adrenal (HPA) axis. The HPA axis is the coordinated system of the three primary endocrine tissues (glands) that mediates our response to stress; in other words, the HPA axis is the "machinery" that helps the body "do its thing" when stress occurs.

So far, everything is perfectly normal: Stress happens and the body reacts immediately (alarm phase) to get things moving, and then works on a more long-term basis (resistance phase) to restore balance. The problems start to occur when we ask the body to react too often (too much alarm) or with excessive exuberance (too much resistance), both of which lead us down the path of having elevated cortisol levels. Under these circumstances, when stress is repeated or constant, cortisol levels go up and stay up, causing a third phase of the general adaptation syndrome that is often referred to as *over-*

load. In this overload stage, bodily systems start to break down and our risk for chronic disease skyrockets. This is when we begin to see problems associated with weight gain, immune-system suppression, depression, anxiety, lack of energy, and inability to concentrate. If the overload phase lasts for a prolonged period of time, we can find ourselves in a serious situation, characterized by gastrointestinal ulceration, widespread tissue dysfunction, and profound metabolic derangement.

ACUTE VERSUS CHRONIC STRESS

This academic discussion of the various stages of the stress response in a bunch of lab rats is all very interesting (really!), but you're probably asking yourself, "What does this mean for me?" Well, it could mean a great deal—depending on how your own body responds to stress, and whether that stress is encountered acutely or chronically. First, let's take a look at what happens inside the body when stress hits. The body's initial response to a perceived acute stressor is the already mentioned fight-or-flight response that we've lived with since the caveman days. When stress hits, the body's energy reserves (fat, protein, and carbohydrates) are rapidly mobilized (through catabolic breakdown of tissues) to deal with the stressor. Levels of adrenaline and cortisol increase, while levels of DHEA (dehydroepiandrosterone) and testosterone decrease. (The combined effects of sustained high cortisol and low DHEA/testosterone lead to muscle loss and fat gain—more on that later.)

Common health effects of dealing with acute stressors typically include increased heart rate and blood pressure, increased breathing rate, increased body temperature and sweating, feelings of anxiety and nervousness, headaches, heartburn, and irritability; these are the things you'll feel while the hormones and neurotransmitters rage throughout your body. The good news about an acute stressor, however, is that because our energy stores are mobilized to either fight off or get away from the stressor, we can use that energy and heightened alertness to do something good—such as exercise.

Unfortunately, if we can't eliminate or escape from the stressor (or use exercise to fool our body into thinking that we're escaping), then the acute stressor quickly becomes a *chronic* stressor.

As the acute stressor becomes more of a chronic stressor, cortisol levels continue to increase and DHEA/testosterone levels continue to decrease. (There is no rule of thumb for when acute crosses the line into chronic; it differs widely among people.) As mentioned above, the dual effect of high cortisol and low DHEA/testosterone leads to muscle loss and fat gain, but it can also have detrimental effects on bone and other tissues (via accelerated breakdown and delayed repair). Typical symptoms associated with chronic stress may include weight gain, fatigue, fluctuations in blood sugar, increased appetite, carbohydrate cravings, muscle weakness, and reduced immune-system function. The loss of muscle tissue leads to a fall in basal metabolic rate (the number of calories the body burns at rest) and marks the turning point between "early" and "late" chronic stress, sometimes called Stage 2 and Stage 3 stress. The early stages of chronic stress can be considered more of a *hypercatabolic* situation, characterized by accelerated tissue destruction, whereas the later stages put a person into more of a *hypoanabolic* state, where the ability to rebuild vital tissues is impaired. At this later stage, much of the damage has already been done—muscle and bone tissues are weaker, sex drive is reduced (because of low DHEA/testosterone, growth hormone, and sex steroids), and the person enters a vicious cycle of increased appetite, reduced caloric expenditure, and accelerated fat accumulation.

Ohio University scientists have suggested that the nature of our modern society often makes chronic stress inescapable. In research studies, they have shown overall exposure to cortisol to be significantly related to the degree of "daily hassles" (more hassles lead to more cortisol) as well as to age (higher age = higher cortisol) and to hours slept (less sleep = more cortisol). Researchers in Boston have suggested that acute or chronic psychological stress is a primary cause not just of cortisol overexposure, but also of inflammatory diseases, including insulin resistance, diabetes, obesity, and heart disease. Inflammation and abdominal fat accumulation are inextricably linked, with cortisol, HSD, and cytokines such as IL-6 working together to promote fat storage in a "chicken-and-egg" scenario. (Cytokines are a class of proteins that play a central role in the immune response. Their presence is a marker for inflammation.) These cellular signals lead to obesity, which leads to inflammation, which leads to more obesity. We know that weight loss leads to a fall in markers of inflammation and to a fall in cortisol exposure, and that controlling stress can lead to reduced appetite and weight loss—so it seems that the chicken/egg scenario can run both ways if you know how to nudge the cycle in the right direction.

The bottom line here is that the body is able to deal with acute stress, and it can do so with great effectiveness as long as the acute stress is dealt with *before* it progresses into the chronic stages. How? By exercising. As the Nike ads used to say about exercise, "Just do it!"—because doing it will be your best hedge against acute stress slipping into the realm of chronic stress (more on the uses and benefits of exercise is presented in Chapters 7 and 9).

But now let's get real. If we all had the time, resources, and inclination to "Just do it" on a regular basis, there would be a lot fewer people reading this book (or at least a few more reading it while walking or running on their treadmills). However, the reality is that most of us (this author included) cannot simply drop what we are doing and run off to "do it" (exercise, that is) at a moment's notice. So we miss a few (or more than a few) exercise sessions, our acute stressors "build up" in a sense, and we slowly slip into the initial stages of chronic stress.

INDIVIDUAL RESPONSES TO STRESS

Okay, so now you know that stress exerts a disruptive influence on the body and that one of its effects is an increase in the release of cortisol. It is important to note, however, that a huge difference exists between people in their ability to tolerate a given amount of stress. Some people can simply "take" a greater load of stress before they begin to break down. That said, even some of the toughest and most "stress-resistant" individuals on the planet, such as Marine Corps recruits, will still succumb to the adverse effects of stress. In one study, military recruits were subjected to five days of extreme exercise, starvation, and sleep deprivation. Not surprisingly, due to the stressful nature of this training, cortisol levels went up and performance deteriorated. The researchers also found that even after five days of rest and refueling, cortisol levels still had not returned to normal—demonstrating the fact that no matter how tough and stress-resistant you think you may be, even *you* have a breaking point.

In another study, this one of Swedish factory workers, differences in the stress response were compared between men and women. The researchers showed that although both male and female workers endured similar levels of stress while at work, stress levels in men fell off quickly when they left work. In contrast, stress levels among the female workers tended to either remain the same or even increase when they left work—suggesting that the women continued to be exposed to high levels of stress hormones while they looked after their family and household responsibilities (so much for gender equality).

Stress researchers frequently study competitive athletes. For obvious reasons, athletes are extremely interested in balancing the "dose" of stress they deliver to their bodies with the amount of recovery necessary for optimal performance. Counteracting the muscle-wasting and fat-gaining effects of prolonged cortisol exposure becomes a large part of maximizing performance gains while minimizing the risk for injury. For many athletes, the delicate balance between training and recovery poses a significant dilemma: To go fast, you have to train hard, but training too hard without adequate recovery will just make you slow, because you'll be tired or get hurt. Athletes who excel are those who are most adept at balancing the three primary components of their program: training, diet, and recovery. A phenomenon known as *overtraining syndrome* has been linked to chronic cortisol exposure—exactly the same situation that we all face in our battle with daily stressors. Although chronic over-training is easy to recognize by its common symptoms of constant fatigue, mood fluctuations, and reduced mental and physical performance (sound familiar?), it may be difficult to detect in its earlier stages—just like the early stages of stress. Therefore, competitive athletes, like each of us, need to become adept at balancing *exposure* to stress with *recovery* from stress in order to approach the optimal physical and mental performance they (and we) are looking for.

IS THERE A "WEAKER SEX" WHEN IT COMES TO STRESS?

Researchers at the Johns Hopkins School of Medicine, in Baltimore, have studied gender differences in stress response; they have found that men tend to respond to psychological stress with more "HPA axis response" while women have a greater "hormonal reaction" to stress. This suggests that men are much more likely to experience cardiovascular side effects (such as high blood pressure and heart attacks) to chronic stress, whereas women may be more likely to succumb to depression or anxiety in the face of chronic stress. That said, there are obviously a wide range of personal and individual differences between different men and different women —so it is impossible to say that all men respond to stress in one way and all women respond to stress in another way.

Scientists at Brandeis University, in Boston, have shown that the quality of one's marital relationship can either exacerbate or alleviate some of the mental stress associated with a stressful job. Those individuals with both high levels of work stress and high levels of marital stress exhibited a flattened cortisol rhythm (suggestive of chronic stress), elevated blood pressure, and suppressed immune function. In a series of related experiments, public-health researchers in London have shown that being "overcommitted" to your work increases stress levels, elevates cortisol exposure by an average of 22 percent, and leads to a higher degree of abdominal obesity.

SUMMARY

That's the general overview of the stress response. Acute stress that is followed by adequate adaptation leads to optimal long-term health. On the other hand, chronic stress that is followed by insufficient adaptation leads to metabolic disturbances, tissue breakdown, and chronic disease.

We all know that stress is "bad" for us—even our grandmothers knew this and their grandmothers before them. But why? The next chapter outlines some of the latest scientific theories and medical evidence suggesting that a large part of the detrimental effects of chronic stress on health may be due to the primary stress hormone: cortisol.

CHAPTER 3

All About Cortisol, the Master Stress Hormone

If you've been paying attention throughout the first two chapters, then you already know the basic relationship between stress and cortisol. For those who missed it, stress makes cortisol levels go up. You also understand that cortisol can be both a "good thing" and a "bad thing," depending on how much cortisol is present in the body and how long it "hangs around." In very general terms, cortisol turns "bad" when you either have too much of it or are exposed to it on a regular basis. The discussion that follows provides a closer look at the dynamics of cortisol metabolism.

THE ENDOCRINE SYSTEM

The vast network of hormones and glands in the body is known as the *endocrine system*. This system is made up of specialized tissues (glands) that play an integral part in our overall response to stress. Through our senses of sight, sound, smell, and even our thoughts, the brain collects information and uses both the nervous system and the endocrine system to respond to what it "observes" in the environment. When we encounter a stressor, whether through our physical or our psychological senses, the endocrine system jumps into action to set things right. Through the coordinated actions of two glands in the brain, the hypothalamus and the pituitary, along with another set of glands that sit just above the kidneys, the adrenal glands, stress causes a cascade of hormonal signals to be set into motion. These hormonal signals involve cortisol, epinephrine (adrenaline), norepinephrine, and numerous intermediary hormones that interact to help regulate important aspects of physiology, such as cardiovascular function, energy metabolism, immune-system activity, and brain chemistry.

THE ADRENAL GLANDS

The two adrenal glands are located just above the kidneys (see Figure 3.1). Each adrenal gland is made up of two parts: the inner medulla, which produces adrenaline, and the outer cortex, which produces cortisol and aldosterone, another steroid hormone that is important in salt/water balance and blood pressure. Cortisol and other glucocorticoids are secreted in response to stimulation of the adrenal glands by adrenocorticotropic hormone (ACTH, also known as *corticotropin*) from the pituitary gland. Secretion of ACTH is under the control of another hormone from the hypothalamus called *corticotropin-releasing hormone* (CRH).

It is easy to see how closely the central nervous system is linked with the endocrine (hormone) system. The brain perceives stress; it responds by secreting CRH from the hypothalamus in the brain; CRH stimulates the pituitary gland (also in the brain) to secrete ACTH; and ACTH travels to the adrenal glands (on top of the kidneys) to stimulate cortisol production.

Cortisol levels typically fluctuate in a fairly rhythmic fashion throughout the day, with the highest levels present in the morning and the lowest present at night. It is important to note, however, that cortisol rhythms can be disrupted by a wide variety of factors, such as emotional and physical stress, inadequate sleep, and various illnesses.

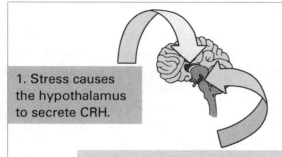

1. Stress causes the hypothalamus to secrete CRH.

2. CRH travels to the pituitary gland and causes secretion of ACTH into the blood.

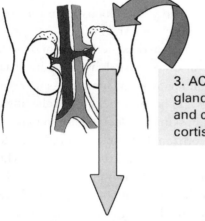

3. ACTH reaches the adrenal glands (above the kidneys) and causes secretion of cortisol (the "stress hormone").

CORTISOL

4. Chronically elevated cortisol levels lead to adverse effects on diverse body systems, including muscle and bone loss, fat gain, elevated blood sugar, high blood pressure, suppressed immune-system function, and changes in memory and mood.

CRH = corticotropin-releasing hormone

ACTH = adrenocorticotropic hormone (also known as corticotropin)

Figure 3.1: The hormonal cascade caused by stress

WHAT IS CORTISOL?

Cortisol, also known as *cortisone* and *hydrocortisone*, is a steroid hormone produced in the adrenal glands in response to stress. As such, cortisol is often referred to as the primary "stress hormone." In the body, cortisol is needed in order to maintain normal physiological processes during times of stress; without cortisol, as discussed in earlier chapters, the body would be unable to respond effectively to stress. Without cortisol, that lion charging at us from the bushes would cause us to do little more than wet our pants and stand there staring (not good). With an effective cortisol metabolism, however, we are primed to run away or do battle, because cortisol secretion releases amino acids (from muscle), glucose (from the liver), and fatty acids (from adipose tissue) into the bloodstream for use as energy. So cortisol is "good"—right? Yes. And no.

Synthetic forms of cortisol, such as dexamethasone and prednisone, are used to treat a wide variety of conditions. They are usually prescribed for their anti-inflammatory and immune-suppressing properties. Cortisol-like drugs can be quite helpful in relieving excessive inflammation in certain skin disorders (Chattem makes an anti-itch skin cream called Cortizone), as well as in inflammatory diseases such as arthritis, colitis, or asthma (the inhalers for which contain corticosteroids). During organ transplantation, cortisol-like drugs are used to suppress the body's immune response, thereby helping to reduce the chance of the body's rejecting the newly transplanted organ. Cortisol-like drugs are also used as replacement therapy for people who have lost function of their adrenal glands (Addison's disease). So, again, cortisol is a "good thing"—right? Yes, but only at certain levels and for a certain period of time.

WHAT DOES CORTISOL DO?

Cortisol has diverse and highly important effects on regulating aspects of all parts of the body's metabolism of glucose, protein, and fatty acids. The functions of cortisol are also particularly important when it comes to controlling mood and well-being, immune cells and inflammation, blood vessels and blood pressure, and in the maintenance of connective tissues such as bones, muscles, and skin. Under conditions of stress, cortisol normally maintains blood pressure and limits excessive inflammation. Unfortunately, many people's adrenal stress response overreacts by secreting too much cortisol—with devastating consequences.

Cortisol and related corticoids are also known as *glucocorticoids*, a term that, as was pointed out in the preceding chapter, is derived from early scientific observations that these hormones are intimately involved in glucose metabolism. Cortisol is known to stimulate several metabolic processes that collectively serve to increase concentrations of glucose in blood.

These effects include stimulation of gluconeogenesis (conversion of amino acids into glucose), mobilization of amino acids from muscle tissues (to serve as the raw material in gluconeogenesis), inhibition of glucose uptake in muscle and adipose (fat) tissue (which further increases blood-sugar levels), and stimulation of fat breakdown in adipose tissue. Unfortunately, the fatty acids released by lipolysis (fat breakdown) have a detrimental effect on health, as they reduce cellular sensitivity to insulin, a condition that can be a precursor to diabetes. Cortisol also has potent anti-inflammatory and immunosuppressive properties—both of which are important in regulating normal responses of the immune system.

THE GOOD, THE BAD, AND THE UGLY OF CORTISOL METABOLISM

The preceding few paragraphs certainly place cortisol in a positive light by focusing on the "good" aspects of cortisol metabolism—and they outline exactly what we would expect from a "normal" pattern of cortisol metabolism (that is, in a perfect world). In that perfect world, cortisol metabolism would look something like this: A stressor is encountered, the endocrine system is activated, the stressor is dealt with, and the stress response is ended. All in all, a very simple reaction. However, when the endocrine system becomes either *over*activated or *chronically* activated (on a regular or repeated basis), the result can be an overall dysregulation of the endocrine system that can lead to a gradual and progressive deterioration of general health and a worsening of existing conditions.

So why even have a stress response if it causes so many problems? Good question. Back in our "caveman" days, this stress response was a vital survival technique—and *not* having such a response would have meant that we were easy prey for saber-toothed tigers and other predators. To repeat how all this works (because it is such an important part of understanding the health problems that arise from chronic stress), the stress response involves a brief increase in energy levels, hormone levels, and ability for forceful muscle contraction—otherwise known as the *fight-or-flight* mechanism. The phrase "fight or flight" means just what it says: It prepares the body to deal with the stressor by either attacking it or running away from it. Unfortunately, even in these modern times, when we're faced with a "benign" stressor, such as a project deadline or a traffic jam (these may be irritating, but they're not going to swallow you like the aforementioned tiger), our bodies undergo the very same metabolic stress changes—which can lead us down the path to increased disease risks.

Under normal circumstances, the body does a pretty good job of controlling cortisol secretion and regulating the amount of cortisol in the bloodstream—but not always (more on this later). Normal cortisol metabolism follows a circadian rhythm (see Figure 3.2)—meaning that levels tend to follow a twenty-four-hour cycle—with the highest cortisol levels typically observed in the early morning (about 6:00 to 8:00 A.M.) and the lowest levels in the wee hours of the morning (about midnight to 2:00 A.M.). Cortisol levels usually show a rapid drop between 8:00 A.M. and 11:00 A.M., and they undergo a continued gradual decline throughout the day. After reaching the lowest levels at around 2:00 A.M., cortisol levels begin to rise again to help us wake up and prepare for another stressful day.

It is interesting to note that people who work the graveyard shift for prolonged periods of time (more than a year) undergo al-

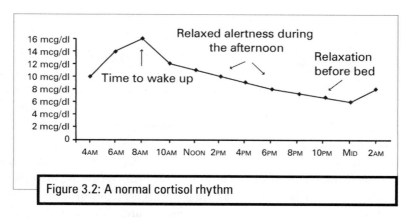

Figure 3.2: A normal cortisol rhythm

terations in their "cortisol clocks." Their cortisol levels are lowest during the day, when people who work this shift get their deepest sleep, and their levels start to rise again in the late afternoon to early evening when they must get up and get ready for their night work. This is exactly opposite from the pattern we see in people with "normal" work schedules. However, it is important to note that most shift workers (those who pick up an occasional late shift now and again) show no such adaptation in cortisol metabolism. For these people, the additional late shift merely disrupts sleep patterns and keeps cortisol elevated when it should be falling.

The "normal" range for blood cortisol levels is fairly wide, 6–23 mcg/dl (micrograms per deciliter), but these levels can vary tremendously in response to stress, illness, and even following meals, each of which increases cortisol levels. Blood cortisol measurements are also affected by the time of day at which they are collected, because cortisol levels are usually high in the morning and low at night. Urinary levels of cortisol have an even wider range of "normal" values (10–100 mcg/dl over twenty-four hours), but because urine samples are collected over a twenty-four-hour period, this measurement at least avoids the issue of the large circadian (daily) variations in cortisol levels seen in blood measurements. The problem with measuring cortisol levels in urine is that the range of normal values is huge. Cortisol levels can also be elevated by estrogen hormone therapy, exercise, pregnancy, depression, anxiety, and even by the intake of mild stimulants such as ephedra (used for weight loss) or caffeine (as little as two to three cups of coffee will elevate cortisol levels).

Now, for some of the *bad* aspects of cortisol metabolism. If the above information makes you think that your "normal" cortisol levels are at risk for becoming elevated, then you're not alone. In fact, with today's Western lifestyles being defined by our fast-paced, low-sleep, fast-food habits, it would be surprising to find people who did *not* experience elevated cortisol levels on a regular basis. "So what," you say? You're not afraid of no stinkin' cortisol? Well, you should be. To reemphasize yet another point that bears repeating from the earlier chapters, here's why: There is very good scientific and medical evidence to show that chronically elevated cortisol levels are associated with obesity, hypertension, diabetes, fatigue, depression, moodiness, irregular menstrual periods, decreased sex drive, and Alzheimer's disease.

Whenever our bodies are exposed to a stressor, cortisol springs into action to increase levels of fat and sugar in the bloodstream, which can be used by the brain and muscles to deal with the stressor. Normally, cortisol levels are quickly depleted following the stress response. Unfortunately, the way our bodies were designed to deal with stress (fight or flight) is not the way we deal with stress in our modern world, where we simply try to ignore the stress hormones pulsing through our bodies. This scenario means that our bodies are unable to deplete their stores of stress hormones—which induces even more stress and stimulates an even more pronounced secretion of cortisol.

Because our bodies were meant to deal only with immediate short-term exposure to stress hormones, this chronic long-term exposure to cortisol can quickly lead to breakdowns in the body's metabolic control systems. Most of the problems associated with elevated cortisol levels have their origins in a disrupted metabolism, causing elevations in blood sugar, cholesterol, blood pressure, and body-fat levels. This cluster of related metabolic disturbances is termed the *metabolic syndrome,* or sometimes *syndrome* X. Many people with syndrome X are easily recognizable because of their accumulation of abdominal body fat (they look apple-shaped) and their high waist-to-hip ratio (WHR). Research has clearly shown that the higher a person's WHR (the bigger one's waist circumference compared to his or her hip circumference), the higher his or her risk for developing syndrome X. An optimal WHR is usually considered anything under 0.8 (meaning a smaller waist than hip circumference), while anything over 0.85 puts a person at risk for syndrome X (more on syndrome X is presented in Chapter 6).

Recall from Chapter 1 (in the section titled "Stress and Disease") how one of the most notable effects of chronically elevated cortisol levels is an increase in appetite and cravings for certain foods. These cravings tend to be for calorie-dense sweets and salty snacks—and this illustrates in one more way the fact that human beings were simply not meant to carry around constant disturbances in our stress response (chronic stress); we were built to respond to stress quickly and then to have those stress hormones dissipate immediately. When our bodies are exposed to wave after wave of the stress that comes from modern lifestyles, our bodies gradually begin to break down. Animals simply don't normally harbor chronic stress the way humans do.

THE CATABOLIC EFFECTS OF CHRONICALLY ELEVATED CORTISOL

Too much cortisol for too long a period of time leads from the merely "bad" to the downright "ugly" aspects of cortisol overexposure. This ugly phase is characterized by widespread tissue destruction and system breakdown (also referred to as *catabolism*), such as muscle loss, bone loss, immune-system suppression, and brain shrinkage.

For example, very brief exposure to cortisol, such as during periods of acute fight-or-flight stress, causes an initial stimulation of immune-system activity and mental ability (good things if you are trying to evade a predator). Even this initial stimulatory effect of cortisol can *over*activate the immune system in some people, leading to allergies, asthma, and a variety of autoimmune diseases such as rheumatoid arthritis, lupus, and fibromyalgia (all of which are known to be triggered by stressful events). On the other hand, a more chronic, longer-term exposure to cortisol has the opposite effect, causing immune cells to die and *in*activating our immune-system protection system. (These phenomena are explained in more detail in Chapter 6, where we see the wide-ranging health effects of chronic stress.)

CORTISOL IS ONLY ONE PIECE
OF THE PUZZLE

From the preceding discussion, it is obvious that cortisol plays a pivotal role in the stress response and how the biochemistry of stress can work with you or against you—yet cortisol is only one piece of the relationship between stress and disease. As previous sections have shown, the length and severity of your body's response to a given stressor can determine your degree of cortisol exposure: high, low, or medium, and flat or fluctuating. In turn, cortisol's counterregulatory hormone, testosterone, must also be in constant flux, ideally rising to counteract the catabolic effects of elevated cortisol. Unfortunately, chronic cortisol overexposure tends to *reduce* testosterone levels—an effect that is doubly bad for maintaining mood, muscle mass, and metabolic rate, so weight gain is virtually inevitable in the face of high cortisol and low testosterone. (We'll concern ourselves with testosterone in much greater detail in Chapter 5.)

In addition to the counteracting effects between catabolic cortisol and anabolic testosterone (an interplay that occurs in both men and women), we need to be especially concerned about the activity of a little-known "fat-storing" enzyme located deep within fat cells. This enzyme, known as 11 beta-hydroxysteroid dehydrogenase-1 (11 beta-HSD, or HSD for short), causes inactive cortisol (cortisol that has done its job and has been deactivated by the body) to become "reactivated" into active cortisol *within* individual fat cells. This is a particularly big problem for *abdominal* fat cells because it is fat cells in this part of the body that respond so strongly to the "fat-storage" signal of cortisol. More cortisol means more fat storage—

and when that cortisol signal is coming from right within each individual fat cell, the fat-storage response is particularly strong. The obvious problem with this HSD effect is that no matter how good you get at avoiding stressful events, or at managing your stress levels, or even at controlling your body's stress response, the resulting low cortisol levels in your blood can still be amplified by HSD to become high cortisol levels within your fat cells (and also in your liver cells, which spells problems for diabetes risk). The next chapter (Chapter 4) goes into some detail about the role of the HSD enzyme as an amplifier of "local" cortisol concentrations within individual cells (as opposed to "systemic" cortisol levels within the blood) and how modulation of HSD activity can add a valuable dimension to our attempts to live in a stressful twenty-first-century world.

SUMMARY

So there you have an overview of the "good, bad, and ugly" aspects of cortisol metabolism. The "good" includes such effects as cortisol's anti-inflammatory benefits, which are great to have, but only for a short period of time in very specific situations. But we all have stress—maybe a lot of stress—and those of us who endure repeated stress, or have hectic lifestyles, or are dieting, or sleep less than eight hours per night are likely to have chronic stress—and chronically elevated cortisol levels. This is when the "bad" aspects of cortisol begin to appear, as metabolic changes that include elevated blood sugar, increased appetite, accelerated weight gain, reduced sex drive, and severe fatigue. Left untreated, these conditions can lead to truly "ugly" problems such as muscle and bone loss, immune-system breakdown, and brain shrinkage.

Whether or not our stress responses and our cortisol exposure ever progress from good to bad to ugly is complicated by the complex interactions of cortisol with testosterone and the HSD enzyme to continually increase cellular cortisol levels. Given the above information, it is vitally important for each of us to approach "cortisol control" as a primary focus

(cont'd.)

for achieving long-term health and well-being. The coming chapters deal with HSD (Chapter 4), testosterone (Chapter 5), and the relationship between stress, cortisol, and disease (Chapter 6). The information in these chapters will help set the stage for you to make meaningful steps toward improving how you feel, how you look, and your risk profile for certain diseases.

. . . .
.
.
.

CHAPTER 4

HSD: The Body's
"Fat Storage" Enzyme

O ne of the complicating factors in the stress/cortisol/fat relationship is a little enzyme deep within fat cells called HSD—
short for 11 beta-hydroxysteroid dehydrogenase-1. (Aren't
you glad we can just call it HSD?) HSD functions to convert inactive cortisol (called corti*sone*) back into active corti*sol*, which then
functions as a potent fat-storage signal within fat cells, especially
abdominal fat cells (those in the belly region). Recent research tells
us that HSD activity is higher in abdominal fat cells than it is in
fat cells in other parts of the body—which may be the reason why
cortisol exposure is associated with higher levels of fat in the abdominal region as compared to fat levels in other parts of the body,
such as the thighs or buttocks.

WHAT IS HSD AND WHAT DOES
IT HAVE TO DO WITH CORTISOL?

HSD is located within almost every cell in the body, but its highest
levels are found in adipose (fat) tissue, liver tissue, and brain tissue. Within all the cells in each of these kinds of tissue, HSD is referred to as a "membrane-bound microsomal enzyme"—meaning it

is attached to the membrane of a structure called the endoplasmic reticulum that resides inside of cells. Because of its position inside each cell, HSD can force the cells to "see" or be exposed to high levels of cortisol, even when blood levels of cortisol are perfectly normal. This effect has led many stress researchers to refer to HSD as a "local amplifier" of cortisol exposure, because no matter what a person's systemic (blood) levels of cortisol look like (low, medium, or high), a highly active HSD enzyme will force each individual cell to be exposed to a high level of cortisol—from the inside! It is a bit like trying to avoid the air pollution outdoors by staying in your house—but HSD sabotages your efforts because it acts like a window fan to suck the bad air into the house and concentrate the pollution there. Yuck!

For many years we have known that obesity is associated with increased cortisol exposure, *but* this relationship was not always a consistent link between obesity and elevated blood levels of cortisol. In some studies, people with high stress and lots of abdominal stress fat had normal or low levels of cortisol in their blood (or urine or saliva), indicating that there was no systemic cortisol overexposure. What we now know is that certain enzymes are dysregulated in obesity—most notably the HSD enzymes in fat tissue—effectively leading to a "high" cortisol level within fat cells at all times. Unfortunately, this means that no matter how good you are at controlling your stress response and, thus, the level of cortisol in your *blood,* you could still have high levels of cortisol within your fat cells because of a high HSD activity.

Don't misunderstand me here. The overall level of cortisol exposure throughout your body (i.e., systemically) is still as important as it ever was, but we understand now that blood levels of cortisol are only half the story—and it is cortisol levels *inside* your cells that represent the other half. In general, higher levels of abdominal fat and total body fat are associated with higher total levels of cortisol in the body. A number of researchers have found that different distributions of fat accumulation are associated with specific changes in cortisol metabolism. Increased abdominal HSD activity, which causes increased generation of active cortisol from inactive cortisone, is generally associated with higher amounts of abdominal fat. This "local" or "peripheral" metabolism of cortisol has rejuvenated the long-standing hypothesis that cortisol contributes to abdominal fat accumulation—and the potency of HSD (how active it is) has emerged as the key.

For decades, research has shown that elevated levels of cortisol lead to more body fat and problems with blood-sugar control. The relationship has always looked relatively clear-cut: More stress leads to more cortisol, which leads to more body fat. In recent years, however, these links have become less straightforward; research findings have shown plenty of people with high stress and high cortisol levels—yet no obesity. Research has also shown people who are overweight—yet have low stress or normal cortisol levels. What's going on? Shouldn't these stressed-out people be getting fat? Not always. Shouldn't these overweight folks, especially those with lots of abdominal "stress" fat, have very high cortisol levels? Not always.

Although the link between stress and cortisol is mostly a direct one (more stress = more cortisol production), and the link between cortisol and abdominal fat is also pretty clear (more cortisol = more belly fat), the picture gets more complicated when we start to talk about *individual* stress levels and *individual* cortisol exposure and *individual* body fat levels.

Researchers from the University of Helsinki, in Finland, have shown that cortisol causes fat accumulation in specific sites most likely to be associated with insulin resistance (prediabetes). These sites are abdominal fat tissue and the liver—and fat accumulates in these areas because of the activity of HSD. Higher activity of HSD means a higher rate of fat storage and a faster accumulation of fat stores. In abdominal areas, a high HSD activity leads to a rounder waistline, while in the liver it means a higher risk for diabetes.

Researchers in Berlin, Germany, have suggested that the regulation of cortisol levels within cells by HSD is *just as important* as cortisol levels in the plasma. This means that the adrenal glands are not the only place in the body for "production" of cortisol; fat calls can produce their own fat-storing cortisol via reactivation of inactive cortisol by the HSD enzyme. This leads to higher cortisol levels within fat cells and a further increase in fat storage and the size of fat cells. Overall, according to the German scientists, it is this mechanism of "self-production" of cortisol within individual fat cells that may represent the most important pathogenic signal for central (abdominal) obesity.

HSD activity is genetically determined, so a person will have either high, low, or "normal" activity—and thus a corresponding level of cortisol conversion and fat storage. None of the lifestyle factors (stress, exercise, etc.) are known to directly affect HSD activity (except via alterations in other hormones, such as growth hormone), which is what makes the enzyme such a tempting target for the drug companies. (More on this topic appears later in this chapter.)

THE EFFECTS OF HSD
ON OBESITY AND DIABETES

So, as discussed, researchers around the world are beginning to understand not only that high levels of systemic cortisol are certainly bad, but also that it is the levels of cortisol within each individual cell that ultimately determine your risk for abdominal obesity, diabetes, high cholesterol, and high blood pressure—the combination we call the metabolic syndrome.

We are now finding that it is the activity of the HSD enzyme— specifically, how fast it converts inactive cortisone into active cortisol—that determines the rate of fat storage in many people. For example, you could have low stress (or be very good at controlling your stress levels) and therefore have low cortisol levels in your blood, *but* if you had a high HSD activity, then your fat cells would always "see" (or be exposed to) a relatively high level of cortisol. This means your fat cells would always be receiving a potent signal telling them to "store more fat"—so no matter what you did in terms of exercise or diet or stress management, you would always be fighting against your own metabolism. Sound familiar?

In most healthy people, overweight or not, systemic (whole-body) cortisol levels are typically "normal"—but what constitutes a normal cortisol range is extremely wide. If your cortisol levels fell outside of the "normal" range on standard laboratory assessments, then you would be so disabled as to be almost bedridden. Instead, most of us who are able to walk around will have cortisol levels within a normal range, but those levels are still probably a lot higher than they need to be. As described in other parts of this book, your cortisol production is probably far too high if you have any of the "big 3" risk factors: chronic stress, restrained eating (dieting), or sleep deprivation—even if you're considered to be "normal" based on standard laboratory measures. Who wants to be normal? And, if normal means a "normal" level of cortisol overexposure, then forget it.

When cortisol circulates in the bloodstream it is only present for about two hours. After that, the body does a pretty good job of deactivating the cortisol so it cannot do any more damage. If, however, you experience another stressful event (and another and another), then you continually expose yourself to more and more cortisol. But remember, equally important to consider is the cortisol *inside* your cells—the stuff activated by the enzyme HSD—and it is this "tissue specific" form of cortisol that may be the worst of all. Luckily, we know of a wide range of natural substances, from licorice to fruit extracts, that can help to control HSD activity. Some of these are discussed in Chapter 8.

As mentioned, the highest levels of HSD activity are seen in the adipose (fat) tissue, liver, and brain—which may be one reason why chronic stress and cortisol overexposure have such a detrimental effect on obesity (adipose tissue), diabetes (liver), and memory (brain). Within your fat cells, a high level of HSD activity results in a dual signal to both store more fat (called "hypertrophy"—where each fat cell gets bigger and bigger) and to increase their proliferation (called "hyperplasia"—an increase in the number of individual fat cells). If all of this weren't bad enough, research has shown that HSD activity tends to increase with age, resulting in a threefold difference between younger (twenty-something) and older (fifty-something) people—and possibly accounting for our growing waistlines as we age.

A team of Scottish and Swedish researchers from the British Heart Foundation, Swedish Heart and Lung Foundation, and Swedish Medical Research Council has shown that blood cortisol levels are often *not* elevated in all cases of obesity; rather, high "intra-adipose" (within fat cells) cortisol levels may be the main culprit in excessive belly-fat storage. This group of scientists has found that high HSD activity levels are associated with both obesity and with insulin resistance. They have also determined that women between the ages of fifty-three and fifty-seven tended to have higher HSD activity and a higher percentage of total body fat compared to men in the same age range—but the relationship between high HSD and more belly fat was the same for both men and women. Overall, this research indicates that both men and women are susceptible to abdominal weight gain from overactive HSD in their fat cells, but women appear to be at a slightly higher risk (which may further increase during menopause).

Researchers from the National Institutes of Health (NIH) have discovered that HSD activity is significantly higher in people with obesity. These findings support previous reports that have suggested that weight gain in many people is disproportionate to food intake. This is what lots of people report, and it's what we routinely see in the clinic: People gain more weight than what we can account for by their dietary or physical-activity patterns. This suggests, and the NIH researchers confirm, that adipose tissue may have its own set of messengers that signal the fat cells to store more fat, independent of food intake. These tissue-specific signaling patterns have been suspected for over thirty years, but simple measurements of cortisol levels in the blood, urine, or saliva have been reported in obese patients as decreased, increased, and unchanged, creating confusion among researchers and health professionals. Now we know that it is excessive *intracellular* activity of the HSD enzyme that turns low levels of cortisol into one of the most potent fat-storage signals, particularly in abdominal fat cells. By slowing the activity of HSD, even just a little bit, we should be able to reduce its production of active cortisol and thus short-circuit its fat-storing effects.

Researchers from the National Institute of Diabetes have found that increased HSD activity in abdominal fat tissue contributes to the worsening of obesity and insulin resistance (prediabetes). In a series of studies that followed subjects for up to five years (an average of two and a half years across all subjects in the study), this group of scientists was investigating why some previous studies had found systemic cortisol levels to be high or low or normal in obese subjects. They reasoned that something else must be going on to explain obesity rates—and they suspected that although systemic cortisol levels are important, it may be tissue-specific cortisol levels that influence weight gain and the development of obesity. (Recall that "tissue-specific" refers to the cortisol levels *inside* a given cell, such as within an individual fat cell.) Even though previous studies had shown HSD levels and overall activity to be related to fat levels in overweight humans, before this study (published in September 2006), no long-term study had been conducted to definitively link HSD to weight gain. Not only did this latest research find a direct relationship between HSD and abdominal fat gain, but it also found a significant association of HSD activity with changes in body weight over time. It was the first clear evidence proving that the higher one's HSD levels, the higher her or his cellular cortisol levels, and the larger the weight gain s/he will experience over time. The mechanism identified by these scientists went beyond what we already knew about cortisol serving as a "fat-storage" signal for fat cells (i.e., more cortisol = more fat storage); it showed that cortisol is also a potent signal for young fat cells (called "preadipocytes") to grow into mature fat cells (called "adipocytes") and rapidly start storing fat. These researchers stated that HSD activity has "a causative role in promoting obesity and its metabolic consequences."

In an interesting series of metabolism studies, scientists from the Mayo Clinic have shown that cortisol can be released into the blood from tissues other than the adrenal glands. As we've seen, abdominal adipose tissue (belly fat) has been identified as a tissue that can create its own supply of cortisol (leading to weight gain). In addition, the liver and other internal organs can also produce a supply of cortisol that can have health effects throughout the body, including increasing the risk of obesity. Writing in the *Journal of the American Diabetes Association*, the Mayo scientists confirmed that the liver and related internal organs converted a large proportion of inactive cortisol into active cortisol via the HSD enzyme—and that the total amount of cortisol produced (or "reactivated") was "equal to if not greater than" the amount produced by the adrenals. Think of it—you could be calm as a cucumber, perfectly managing your stress and cortisol production from the adrenal glands, but you are still overexposed to cortisol because your liver and fat cells are producing cortisol on their own! The researchers went on to calculate that the adrenals, fat cells, and liver all contribute about one-third each of total body cortisol—meaning that your yoga class as a stress-management tool is only influencing about a *third* of your total cortisol exposure.

Researchers from the University of Birmingham, in England, have some especially depressing news for people who are trying to lose weight by extreme dieting. Studying the metabolic effects of a very low calorie diet (eight hundred calories per day) for ten weeks, they found that the stress of the diet significantly increased cortisol levels throughout the body, but also increased HSD activity within fat cells by 3.4 times. This indicates not only that diets are stressful (you already knew that), but also that your fat cells are fighting against you! As you struggle to lose weight, your fat cells *increase* their HSD activity, leading to more cortisol, a stronger signal to store fat, and a gradual return to your prediet body weight. I could not agree more with the researchers' concluding remark that "inhibition of HSD may be a novel therapeutic strategy" for treating diabetes and obesity.

Scottish hormone researchers have recently described the link between elevated HSD activity and abdominal obesity in both stressed and nonstressed situations. We know that many cases of overweight and obesity occur with normal (nonelevated) cortisol levels. In these cases, as described throughout this chapter, it may be that elevated activity of the HSD enzyme is to blame. Indeed, these researchers describe an elevation of HSD levels and activity in human fat cells that may support a disrupted metabolism leading to abdominal fat gain, whether or not stress or cortisol levels are elevated. In another scientific report, this same research group outlines the benefits associated with inhibiting HSD activity as a novel strategy to lower intracellular cortisol levels, without affecting circulating cortisol levels and overall ability to respond to stress. Early experiments in humans show that inhibiting HSD activity allows a normal stress response to occur when it needs to (i.e., when you encounter something stressful), but reduces the effects of excessive stress in fat tissue and brain tissue, and also reduces metabolic effects related to diabetes risk.

According to scientists in the Division of Cardiovascular Medicine at the University of Arkansas, the epidemic of abdominal obesity and the metabolic syndrome in the United States and around the world "may be a stress response, with an underlying abnormality in the enzyme 11 beta-hydroxysteroid dehydrogenase." The researchers go on to lament the fact that there are no pharmaceuticals currently available for the inhibition or control of HSD activity (while observing that drug companies are rapidly inventing synthetic chemicals for just this purpose). What they fail to note is that a variety of natural controllers of HSD activity are available now as dietary supplements (see Chapter 8).

THE PHARMACEUTICAL RUSH
TO BLOCK HSD

Researchers from the National Institutes of Health (NIH) have shown that too much cortisol can lead to a wide range of "modern" diseases, including anxiety, insomnia, memory problems, depression, fatigue, diabetes, muscle loss, osteoporosis, hypertension (high blood pressure), cancer (immune suppression), and especially weight gain and obesity. No surprise there. Based on the latest re-search, however, these same NIH researchers have also suggested that the use of HSD inhibitors "could be useful in the treatment of these diseases, including cognitive dysfunction in elderly men and patients with type 2 diabetes mellitus." As the NIH researchers note, "the pharmaceutical industry is rigorously searching for, de-veloping, and/or testing HSD inhibitors for the treatment of a host of human disorders such as obesity, metabolic syndrome, diabetes, depression, osteoporosis, etc."

Reducing the activity of HSD is certainly a hot area of research within the pharmaceutical industry because such an effect would lead to decreased fat storage within abdominal fat cells (by reduc-ing HSD activity within adipose tissue), as well as a better control of blood sugar and a lower risk of diabetes (by reducing HSD activ-ity within liver cells).

Indeed, just about every major pharmaceutical company in the world is hard at work developing synthetic controllers of HSD, be-cause they understand that slowing the activity of this enzyme may be the "Holy Grail" to stopping the epidemic of obesity and diabe-tes around the world. This epidemic is not just an American issue; it is perhaps the most important health concern in every industri-alized country from Europe to Asia. In China, for example, there are already as many overweight people (more than sixty million) as there are in the United States. Of course, China's sixty million overweight people represent a much smaller percentage of its total population than the United States' sixty million overweight folks (roughly 7 percent in China, compared to about 66 percent in the United States). The point is that China's population of overweight people is growing rapidly, and it is already as big a "market" for the drug companies as that in the United States, which is generally considered the fattest land on the planet.

Reducing the body's fat storage via a pharmaceutical inhibi-tion of HSD is one of the most active areas of the pharmaceuti-cal industry's research and patent activity. Most of the major drug makers are getting in on the act, with Amgen (with Swedish biotech company Biovitrum), Pfizer, Merck, Hoffman/LaRoche, and Abbott Labs among the contenders to be the first to market with their synthetic HSD inhibitor. Because of the length of the drug-development process, don't expect to see any of these drugs at a pharmacy near you until sometime after 2010. Within the next five to ten years, however, most stress physiologists expect HSD inhibitors to become the biggest blockbuster drugs of all time because of their unmatched potential to be a breakthrough in the treatment of diabetes and obesity.

If you can't wait until 2010 and beyond to do something about your HSD activity, then the next section, which covers some of the natural options for controlling HSD, may be for you.

CONTROLLING HSD ACTIVITY NATURALLY

Let's recap: More HSD activity means more belly fat, and you don't want that, so you need to control your HSD. In humans, we know from a number of research studies that the down-regulation (slowing the activity) of HSD is protective against weight gain and enhances hepatic (liver) insulin sensitivity, leading to better blood-sugar control.

Until about ten years ago, obesity and weight gain were, in general, attributed largely to overeating and a lack of exercise. In the last decade, however, exciting new findings have greatly increased our knowledge about factors contributing to the pathogenesis of obesity and its subsequent health effects. As discussed throughout this chapter, the enzyme HSD, which is predominantly found in adipose (fat) tissue, liver tissue, brain tissue, and cells of the adrenal gland, is now known to be directly related to obesity rates in animals and humans.

For example, mice with high levels of HSD activity have two to three times higher cortisol levels within their fat cells—but normal levels of cortisol in their blood. This matches the situation in many human test subjects. We know that animals with elevated HSD levels tend to weigh 25 to 35 percent more—and have larger appetites—than animals with normal levels of HSD, with most of the excess fat confined to the belly region. So, again, although cortisol is an important signal for fat storage throughout the body, when it becomes elevated *within* abdominal fat cells it becomes one of the most potent stimulators of excess belly fat—and the metabolic syndrome that follows.

In a series of experiments conducted by researchers from Harvard University, the British Heart Foundation, Merck pharmaceuticals, and a Swedish biotechnology firm, not only has HSD overactivity been identified as a cause of obesity and diabetes, but *reducing* its activity has been shown to reduce belly fat—despite a high-fat and high-calorie diet! As described in the last section, both biotech and pharmaceutical companies have recognized the importance of HSD for obesity and diabetes treatment.

Danish scientists have recently found that higher levels of growth hormone are associated with reduced HSD activity, a finding that may explain some of the primary effects of growth hormone in reducing body fat (especially belly fat) and increasing muscle mass. As we age, growth-hormone levels decline dramatically, setting the stage for HSD activity to increase. Whereas growth hormone (GH) accounts for as much as 10 to 46 percent of the change in HSD activity, we know that HSD activity can also be regulated by other hormones, such as sex steroids (estrogen and testosterone) and thyroid hormones. It follows that because growth hormone inhibits the activity of HSD, when GH levels fall (as they do in aging), HSD activity goes up, and we gain more fat and lose the ability to control blood sugar effectively. We have known for many years that people with low GH levels also suffer from muscle loss and fat gain, but we did not know until recently that the mechanism for these effects was due to a problem with HSD metabolism. This research indicates that it may be even more important to naturally regulate HSD activity as we age.

Increasing the activity of HSD in a mouse will lead to significant weight gain, specifically within the abdominal area, within as little as nine weeks—even when the mouse is restricted to a low-fat diet. How depressing is that? Have you ever felt that your attempts at restricting your diet to lose weight have very little effect at all? It may be that HSD is working overtime in your body to maintain (and increase) your abdominal fat stores. In humans, we see the very same effects that we see in mice, where accumulation of visceral fat depots (belly fat) is highest in individuals with the highest HSD activity.

Although we are now learning that HSD activity can be artificially disrupted or "blocked" with synthetic drugs, we also know that we can do the very same thing with naturally occurring compounds from fruits, vegetables, and herbs. Some of the strongest controllers of HSD activity are found in foods rich in flavonoids, such as apples and onions (quercetin), grapefruit (naringenin), and soybeans (genistein and daidzein). The most potent of the flavonoids for balancing HSD activity are found in the form of substances known as polymethoxylated flavonoids (PMFs) found in oranges (nobiletin and tangeretin), which can be up to three to five times stronger than other flavonoids.

Licorice (from the licorice plant, *Glycyrrhiza glabra*), contains glycyrrhetinic acid (GA), a flavonoid that inhibits HSD. In animal studies, increasing flavonoid consumption by feeding GA for fourteen weeks has been shown to reduce HSD activity by 30 percent, cortisol levels by 34 percent, and body weight by 28 percent—all from including a bit more flavonoids in the rats' drinking water! Unfortunately, GA also raises blood pressure, so it cannot be used long-term to control HSD and block fat storage in humans. However, when GA was studied as a weight-loss agent in humans (taken along with a drug to control the rise in blood pressure), GA led to a dramatic drop in cortisol levels, a significant loss of body weight, and a specific reduction of abdominal fat—with no significant alterations in diet or exercise patterns (just as had happened with the rats).

What this means for you and your personal HSD profile is that consuming more flavonoids should be a major dietary goal. Eating more apples and onions (for quercetin), grapefruit (for naringenin), and soybeans (for genistein and daidzein) can't hurt—and doing so may help provide a small measure of inhibition of HSD activity. That said, I would recommend consuming more dietary sources of these particular flavonoids rather than trying to add higher levels from dietary supplements. For dietary supplementation of HSD-inhibiting flavonoids, it would make more sense to focus on the PMFs because of their significantly higher metabolic potency compared to other dietary flavonoids. However, PMFs come from citrus *peels*, which you're probably not eating very many of. Instead, they have been isolated and made available in the form of supplements. You can read more about PMFs and other natural dietary supplements in Chapter 8.

SUMMARY

I very much wish that cortisol metabolism were really as simple and straightforward as we once thought. Our previous, and overly simplistic, view that "more stress = more cortisol = more belly fat" and "less stress = less cortisol = less belly fat" still holds true in some regards—and reminds us that we certainly do not want to have high levels of systemic cortisol (as described in the last chapter and in more detail in Chapter 6). But our growing understanding of the role of the HSD enzyme in cortisol metabolism *within* individual cells alerts us to the fact that we really need to be focusing simultaneously on controlling cortisol exposure both outside of cells (blood levels caused by high stress and poor lifestyle) *and* inside of cells (caused by overactive HSD and suboptimal levels of GH and testosterone).

CHAPTER 5

Testosterone:
Cortisol's Alter Ego

Because of media reports of athletes abusing anabolic steroids (synthetic versions of testosterone), testosterone has suffered a negative public image that is not deserved. Many people view testosterone as the hormone that causes bulging muscles and aggressiveness, but it is important to understand that these effects are caused by a gross overuse of synthetic testosterone at extreme, megadose levels. When bodybuilders and other athletes inject testosterone and other anabolic steroids to promote freakish muscle growth or enhance performance, they are artificially increasing their testosterone levels to ten, twenty, or even a hundred times normal values. The results of this unnatural testosterone exposure are the clearly unnatural changes in body shape, mood, and metabolism characteristic of professional bodybuilders.

WHAT IS TESTOSTERONE?

In both men and women, testosterone is needed to build muscle and other tissues, including skin, tendons, bones, immune-system components, and to control many aspects of physiology, including blood cell production and metabolism of protein, carbohydrates, and fat from food. A drop in testosterone in men leads to fatigue, a loss of sex drive, and weight gain in the belly—the old potbelly that nobody wants. In women, a drop in testosterone causes the same fatigue and loss of sex drive, and it also induces women's bodies to lose their "hourglass" shape of youth and grow into an apple (or "shot glass") shape via a pattern of abdominal weight gain.

In both sexes, some of the most common effects of low testosterone include:

- Emotional changes (increased anxiety and depression)
- Low sex drive
- Decreased muscle mass
- Reduced metabolic rate
- Increased abdominal fat
- Weak bones
- Back pain
- Elevated cholesterol

Think you might be at risk for low testosterone levels? Answer the questions below to find out:

Have you experienced a recent drop in energy levels?

Do you have a lower sex drive than you used to?

Has your strength or endurance decreased recently?

Do you often get sleepy after eating dinner?

Are you more grouchy or "blue" than normal?

Are you less excited about your life lately?

Has there been any recent deterioration in your work ability?

Has there been any recent deterioration in your ability to play sports or exercise?

The more questions you answered "yes" to, the more likely you are to have suboptimal testosterone levels—and the more important it is for you to take immediate steps to restore your testosterone to normal levels. Why? Because in numerous clinical studies, in both men and women, the benefits of maintaining normal testosterone levels (versus low levels) include:

- Improved mood
- A heightened sense of well-being
- Increased mental and physical energy levels
- Improved sleep quality
- Improved sex drive and performance
- Increased lean body mass and muscle strength
- A decline in fat mass
- Reduced cholesterol levels (with a better ratio of "good" to "bad" forms of cholesterol)

NOT JUST FOR MEN

Testosterone—just for men? Hardly! Often referred to as the "hormone of desire," testosterone is involved in maintaining sex drive, mood, muscle mass, and energy levels in *both* men and women. We have known since the mid-1980s that testosterone is not just a "male" hormone, because it was in 1985 that researchers published the first major study showing that testosterone was vitally important in boosting and maintaining a woman's libido (sexual arousal and desire). More than two decades later, American women still do not have a testosterone product to treat sexual dysfunction or arousal problems, despite the fact that after the age of thirty their testosterone levels start to decrease (just like they do in men). What follows is the very predictable drop in sex drive, loss of muscle mass, reduction in metabolic rate, and decrease in energy levels and mood. What goes up? You guessed it: body weight. And we see the same thing happening in men.

Although women produce only about one-tenth the amount of testosterone that men do, a woman's levels drop by about half by the age of forty-five (compared to the amount she produced at age twenty). In a scientific review by the North American Menopause Society, nine out of ten studies on testosterone in women showed increasing testosterone levels to be effective in improving sexual desire, energy levels, and overall emotional outlook. Unfortunately, despite the results of these research studies, there is no female-specific testosterone treatment available to American women, so either they have to try preparations made for men (which may not be appropriate in terms of dosage) or they have to "deal with" feeling lousy.

Luckily, there exist a variety of natural options for improving the body's release of endogenous testosterone (testosterone that is present naturally). Both men and women can benefit from freeing up the testosterone that is already circulating in the blood but that may be locked up by transporters called "binding hormones."

Most testosterone production in women comes from the ovaries and in men from the testes, but in both genders a substantial amount of testosterone also comes from the adrenal glands—the same gland responsible for cortisol production. During periods of high cortisol production (stress, dieting, and sleep loss), our natural production of testosterone falls. Considering that women produce only about one-tenth the amount of testosterone found in men, any stress-induced drop in testosterone would be expected to affect women as much as or more than most men. The effects of stress in older women are even worse because female testosterone levels peak in the mid-twenties—just as they do in young men—and fall every year thereafter. So the average person is less able to "bounce back" from a stressful event at age forty compared to age twenty.

For women who want to stay lean, strong, healthy, fit, and sexually active, maintaining a youthful testosterone level is just as important as it is for men. In fact, studies published in the *New England Journal of Medicine* have shown that testosterone maintenance in women ages thirty-one to fifty-six yields the very same benefits in sexual function, mood, energy, and overall sense of well-being as those found in studies of men.

MAINTAINING BALANCE:
THE CORTISOL-TO-TESTOSTERONE RATIO

Think you're tough enough to fight stress? Think again. Scientists from the United States Army Research Institute have found that even the most elite combat soldiers are not immune to the detrimental effects of stress. In one training exercise, elite Army officers (the most highly motivated and well-trained troops), when exposed to moderate levels of sleep deprivation, experienced elevated cortisol and reduced testosterone, which led to significant changes in mood such as reduced vigor and increased fatigue, confusion, and depression. This study, and others like it, show us that "being tough" in the face of stress is ridiculous, because your body reacts with a predictable stress response: cortisol up and testosterone down (unless you do something to modulate it).

The balance between levels of cortisol and testosterone is probably even more important than the absolute level of either hormone. From the perspective of achieving peak physical and mental performance, you want to have a relatively low cortisol level and a relatively high testosterone level, a hormonal profile that we would refer to as "anabolic" to suggest fat loss and muscle gain. This is what athletes strive for, but it is also your target for optimal weight loss and long-term health.

Iranian medical researchers have shown that the psychological stress of exams increases cortisol and reduces testosterone levels in both male and female students. And British researchers from the University of Bristol have found that elevated cortisol and reduced testosterone (which we refer to as an elevated C:T ratio) increase the risk of heart disease. The British study, which followed men ages forty-five to fifty-nine for more than sixteen years and was published in the scientific journal of the American Heart Association, also found that the C:T ratio was strongly related to insulin resistance (prediabetes). Researchers in Denmark have confirmed the heart-damaging effects of stress by showing that increased cortisol and reduced testosterone are independently related to an increase in blood-vessel thickening, a significant risk factor for heart disease, in both men and women. Italian researchers have shown that low testosterone is associated not only with weight gain but also with increased levels of "bad" cholesterol, lower levels of "good" cholesterol, insulin resistance (prediabetes), and an overall higher risk of heart disease.

The C:T ratio is studied quite often in athletes, not only because of the performance aspects of cortisol and testosterone but also because athletes represent an ideal "high-stress" situation that can help answer important questions about how humans adapt to chronic stress. For example, physiology researchers from the University of North Carolina have shown a clear negative relationship between cortisol levels and testosterone levels in athletes—meaning that as stress gets higher, cortisol goes up and testosterone drops. Researchers from the University of Connecticut have shown that overtrained athletes have elevated levels of sex hormone–binding globulin (SHBG, which binds testosterone, making it unavailable to the body) and reduced testosterone levels—both of which could be prevented by dietary supplementation.

TESTOSTERONE AND AGING: MENOPAUSE AND ANDROPAUSE

Athlete studies aside, by the time most of us, both men and women, reach our forties, our testosterone levels are about 20 percent lower than they were when we were robust twenty-year-olds. (No wonder we're fatter and more exhausted!) In most people, testosterone levels start to fall by about 10 percent per decade (1 percent per year) after age twenty or thirty. At the same time, our bodies start to produce more SHBG, which "traps" most of the testosterone that still remains in circulation. This is bad because SHBG effectively reduces the body's "bioavailable" levels of testosterone even further.

Around age fifty, women are likely to hit menopause and experience dramatic drops in both estrogen *and* testosterone. While men obviously don't experience menopause, at a similar age they do experience a much larger drop in testosterone levels—a change that is referred to as *andro*pause. During this time of life, when hormone production is falling in both men and women, as many as 30 percent of people will have testosterone levels low enough to cause noticeable symptoms. Some of the clearest signs of a testosterone imbalance are changes in attitude and mood, as well as a loss of energy and sex drive.

Researchers from the Mayo Clinic have documented the fall in testosterone levels to be in the range of 35 to 50 percent by age sixty in healthy men, while researchers on aging from Saint Louis University have shown that testosterone levels fall 47 percent in men from age twenty to age eighty-nine. Dozens of studies show that maintaining testosterone levels at more "youthful" levels (that is, preventing them from dropping with age) is associated with numerous health benefits in both men and women. For example, men and women with low testosterone develop abdominal obesity (belly fat), experience a loss in sex drive (interest and ability), and become depressed (or at least moody). Preventive-medicine specialists from the University of California at San Diego have shown that high levels of stress lead to lower testosterone levels (reduced by 17 percent) and increased rates of depression in men over age fifty. Indeed, it is well described in the scientific and medical literature that men who have low levels of testosterone are more likely to suffer from depression than men with normal testosterone levels. When testosterone levels are brought back to normal, mood also returns to normal.

If you look at testosterone on an overall scale, it is not a "more is better" story, but rather one of "maintaining optimal levels is good" and "falling levels are bad." That is, it's one of overall balance.

TESTOSTERONE AND WEIGHT GAIN

For many people, perhaps the most noticeable side effect of a falling testosterone level will be an expanding waistline. Just as increasing cortisol levels can lead to excess belly fat, so can declining testosterone levels—and when you have both occurring simultaneously (cortisol levels rising and testosterone levels falling), it is virtually inevitable that weight gain will follow.

A study published in 1996 in the *Journal of Clinical Endocrinology and Metabolism* showed that obese women who boosted their testosterone levels lost significantly more abdominal fat and gained more muscle mass compared to women who were given a placebo and whose testosterone levels remained suppressed. This was ten *long* years ago—and still most doctors and health professionals view testosterone strictly as a "male" hormone, when the reality is that while women certainly don't want "male levels" of testosterone, they definitely want to maintain what they have.

The scientific literature that supports the maintenance of normal youthful testosterone levels (versus allowing them to *fall* in the face of stress and aging) is at least as strong as the research in support of maintaining normal youthful cortisol levels (which *rise* in response to stress and aging). Here is a sampling of some of the available studies:

Austrian medical researchers have shown that weight loss from dieting results in a significant reduction in testosterone levels in overweight women. But this effect is largely due to a high level of dieting stress caused by excessive calorie restriction (which elevates cortisol) that is not balanced out by exercise (which could maintain testosterone levels). Researchers from Penn State University have shown that weight loss induced by diet alone leads to a significant drop in testosterone and fat-free mass (muscle)—an effect that can reduce metabolic rate and make weight regain easier.

Scientists from Northwestern University, in Chicago, have shown that weight gain in young men (ages twenty-four to thirty-one) was significantly related to low testosterone levels, with a graded relationship between the lowest testosterone levels and the greatest degree of weight gain. In a related series of studies, researchers at Cornell Medical College, in New York, found that the age-related decrease in testosterone is significantly exacerbated in overweight men with the metabolic syndrome. As testosterone drops, body weight goes up—and the drop in testosterone and the rise in weight are more pronounced in men who have metabolic syndrome than it is in men without. (Men who don't have the condition also gain weight as testosterone drops, but to a less severe degree.)

As part of the Massachusetts Male Aging Study (which followed over seventeen hundred men, ages forty to seventy), researchers from the New England Research Institutes found that overweight men had significantly lower testosterone levels and a greater rate of decline compared to normal-weight men of any age. Endocrine researchers in Venezuela have found that testosterone levels are lower in overweight men ages twenty to sixty and that there is a graded and proportional relationship between low testosterone and weight gain (the fattest men had the lowest testosterone).

Norwegian medical researchers have shown that the lowest levels of testosterone are found in men with the most pronounced central (abdominal) obesity. In addition, those with lower testosterone also had higher blood pressure and increased rates of diabetes. These findings suggest that testosterone may have a protective effect against weight gain and development of diabetes and hypertension.

In a very important study by researchers in aging from the University of Florida, the incidence of low testosterone in a general population of men over age forty-five was estimated to be 38.7 percent. Those with low testosterone were also about twice as likely to be overweight and to have hypertension, high cholesterol, and diabetes.

In a study from researchers at the Albert Einstein College of Medicine, in New York, overweight men were shown to have reduced testosterone levels, with the lowest levels seen in men who continued to gain weight over time (eight years follow-up). Interestingly, the level of testosterone was found to *predict* subsequent weight gain: Lower testosterone related specifically to increased weight gain in the abdominal area.

Australian scientists at the University of Adelaide have shown that testosterone levels decline with aging even in healthy men—and also lead to obesity and metabolic syndrome.

Italian hormone researchers have shown a negative relationship between C:T ratio and obesity in men and women. As stress-related cortisol levels rise, testosterone levels drop in both sexes, leading to weight gain, especially within the abdominal area.

Public-health researchers in Hong Kong have shown that age-related declines in testosterone are associated with increased levels of abdominal fat and higher rates of the metabolic syndrome. In a series of studies, low testosterone levels explained 35 percent of the variance in metabolic syndrome rates (more metabolic syndrome equated with lower testosterone).

Brazilian medical researchers have found low testosterone levels to be strongly associated with weight gain and specifically with higher abdominal fat (waist-to-hip ratio). Norwegian researchers have shown that the lowest testosterone levels are found in subjects with high waist circumference, even when their total level of body fat is rather normal, suggesting that waist circumference (abdominal fat) is the preferred anthropometric measurement to predict testosterone levels (bigger waist = lower testosterone).

Health researchers from Oklahoma State University have demonstrated a direct effect of testosterone on adipose tissues (fat cells) and obesity, showing that testosterone leads to an increase in lipolysis (fat breakdown). Normal testosterone levels lead to a normal distribution of body fat, but as testosterone levels decrease in response to stress and aging, there is a tendency to increase central obesity (gain abdominal fat). In fact, bringing testosterone levels back to within normal ranges in older men and women has been shown to reduce the degree of central obesity.

Researchers at the University of Washington, in Seattle, have shown that among women who lose weight using dietary restriction alone, each 2 percent loss of body weight is associated with a fall in testosterone levels of 10 to 12 percent.

These studies represent only a fraction of the research on the relationship between testosterone, stress, cortisol, and weight gain, but it should be clear to you by now that the failure to maintain a normal C:T balance is an important reason why weight gain (and regain) is so easy for so many people. As we attempt to lose weight, our bodies try to "fight back" by slowing metabolism and conserving body fat through a rise in cortisol levels, a drop in testosterone levels, and a decline in muscle mass and metabolic rate. As a result of these metabolic changes, fat cells lose the "fat-breakdown" signal (testosterone) and receive the "fat-storage" signal (cortisol)—and weight appears (or easily comes back).

MAINTAINING TESTOSTERONE LEVELS NATURALLY

As with other hormones, including cortisol, we know quite clearly that maintaining optimal levels of testosterone—not too high and not too low—is the approach associated with the most dramatic long-term health benefits. In the context of the SENSE Lifestyle Program, keeping cortisol levels "low" and testosterone levels "high" really means maintaining *optimal* values in the face of stress and aging (both of which raise cortisol and lower testosterone).

It is important to keep in mind that one of the most central concepts in the science of endocrinology (the study of hormones) is that hormones tend to work *in concert* with one another to control metabolism. This means that changing two hormones, each by a little bit, is likely to have a better overall effect on a given outcome (such as weight loss) than changing a single hormone by a large amount. In the case of the SENSE program, the last five years have shown us that a small change in cortisol (5 percent reduction) plus a small change in testosterone (5 percent increase) delivers a much more profound change (loss of body fat, increase in energy and mood) than does a large change in cortisol (20 percent reduction) by itself. In our most recent iteration of the SENSE program, the average reduction in the cortisol/testosterone ratio was 15 percent—and participants could not believe how good they felt or how easy it was to drop the fat. (The entire SENSE Lifestyle Program is outlined in Chapter 9.)

In addition, changing multiple hormones by small amounts is also much less likely to lead to side effects and other problems associated with "single-focused" approaches to weight loss. By controlling stress and using supplements to maintain normal cortisol/testosterone levels, we have much better compliance and success rates than programs such as low-carb diets or those relying on stimulant-based herbs. Better results with fewer side effects—I think you would agree that is not a bad approach.

Chapter 8 covers a number of dietary supplements that can help to maintain normal testosterone levels, but there are several other simple techniques that can also help, including getting enough sleep (Chapters 7 and 9), staying physically active, maintaining adequate hydration, and learning to perceive stressful events in the proper context.

In terms of physical activity, we know that virtually all forms of exercise help to elevate testosterone levels in both men and women; endurance exercise works almost as well as lifting weights for maintaining testosterone in most moderate exercisers. Researchers at the University of Texas have shown that not only does inactivity lead to a rapid loss of muscle mass, but when accompanied by high levels of stress and cortisol, muscle loss is accelerated. The good news about exercise is that while it is boosting testosterone, it is also reducing cortisol, via the "destressing" effect of a workout. But the best news of all is that you'll be pleasantly surprised by how little exercise is needed to activate these positive hormonal effects (covered in Chapter 9).

Avoiding dehydration is another way to keep your hormones balanced. Researchers from the University of Connecticut's Human Performance Laboratory demonstrated that cortisol levels were increased by dehydration. In addition, C:T ratio was significantly higher (i.e., elevated C and reduced T), creating a biochemical state that interferes with the balance between anabolism and catabolism, which in this case shifts the body toward fat gain and muscle loss.

Finally, stress researchers from around the world have shown that how we perceive and cope with a given stressor can determine our hormonal response to that stressor. For example, Italian researchers have found that health effects of daily stressful encounters are related to how the stress is perceived. This means you can be exposed to stress, and deal with it appropriately, resulting in only a temporary, healthy rise in cortisol levels. However, if the stress is dealt with inappropriately (for example, if you mentally "revisit" the event over and over), your cortisol levels rise and testosterone levels fall. Likewise, psychology researchers in Spain have shown that when men or women cope with any sort of social "competition," we assess it in such a way that it activates a "psychobiological coping response." The important thing here is that both the significance of the competition and your perception of the amount of control you have over the outcome will influence your biochemical stress response to the situation. More important than winning or losing is the coping pattern you display, thus determining your hormonal changes. Psychologists at the University of Miami use cognitive-behavioral stress management (CBSM) to reduce perceived stress in stressful or competitive situations. Participating in CBSM activities causes cortisol levels to drop and levels of anabolic hormones (like testosterone and DHEA) to rise—effects that typically translate into an improvement in both mood and in immune function.

SUMMARY

It is probably quite apparent to you by now that it is a *balance* between hormones and enzymes that represents the "metabolic sweet spot" you're shooting for. In a perfect world, we would easily maintain the relatively low cortisol and high testosterone levels of our youth, and pesky fat-storing enzymes like HSD would be adequately controlled with liberal and frequent infusions of hot fudge sundaes. Alas, the very process of living and aging (gracefully or not) leads us inexorably toward elevated cortisol, suppressed testosterone, and overactive HSD—all of which combine to make us rounder and softer and more tired and less happy.

Now that you're completely depressed about how different elements of your body's biochemistry gang up to destroy your figure, it's time to throw you off the cliff by outlining

(cont'd.)

the relationship between stress (and the resulting hormone/ enzyme changes) and your risk for most modern diseases. This topic is outlined in Chapter 6, but please don't despair, because Chapters 7 through 9 are where we get into the good news: that you can *do something* to maintain optimal levels of cortisol, testosterone, and HSD—even in the face of a too-stressful existence.

The Relationship Between Stress and Disease

So now you know a bit about how chronic stress leads to elevated cortisol and reduced testosterone levels in the body. This chapter details the next piece of the puzzle: the relationship between cortisol/testosterone ratios and the risk for a wide range of chronic diseases. For the sake of simplicity, when I refer to "elevated cortisol levels" or to "cortisol overexposure," you should assume that I am referring not only to excess cortisol, but also to suboptimal testosterone.

It should come as no big surprise to anybody reading this book that the effects of stress on a person's long-term health can be far-reaching. The medical literature tells us quite clearly that many of the negative conditions associated with a "modern" lifestyle—such as obesity, diabetes, hypertension, insomnia, headaches, ulcers, depression, anxiety, poor memory, and a lower resistance to infections—are all related to high stress levels. Also noteworthy is the consistent finding that people dramatically increase their use of the medical system during times of heightened stress (such as a period of job insecurity) and that there is a tight association between elevated cortisol levels and higher health-care costs. Episodes of illness, doctor visits, and trips to hospital outpatient departments have been shown to double (at least) during high-stress periods when compared to lower-stress periods. We see this same pattern emerge during final-exam week on college campuses, when walk-in health clinics are filled with sick students during their most stressed-out time of the year. Other evidence clearly demonstrates that workers reporting the highest level of perceived stress due to job dissatisfaction, family problems, and personal conflict are the most likely to experience somatic symptoms such as colds, flu, allergies, asthma, and headaches.

METABOLIC CONSEQUENCES OF ELEVATED STRESS LEVELS

Okay, so cortisol is toxic—right? Not so fast. As we know from the previous chapters, cortisol is a vital hormone; without it, the body would be ill prepared to deal with the stresses of daily life. On the other hand, excess cortisol secretion and chronically elevated cortisol levels can lead to a host of related metabolic disturbances and an increased risk for developing a variety of chronic conditions. We touched on many of these effects in the preceding chapters, and they are summarized here in Table 6.1.

Stress-related diseases occur because of an excessive activation of the stress response in the brain and in the endocrine (hormone) system in reaction to common, everyday sources of physical and psychological stress. The various daily stressors to which we are all subjected can disrupt the body's stable balance of temperature, blood pressure, and other functions. Unfortunately, as mentioned before, because the human brain is so well developed, it can also respond to *imagined* stress with the very same stress response that is supposed to be reserved for life-or-death (fight-or-flight) situations. Accordingly, injury, hunger, heat, cold, or worry can trigger the stress response just as would happen if you were running for your life or fighting off an attacker.

In 1999, a team of Swedish researchers showed that exposure to high levels of stress caused a rapid increase in cortisol secretion,

Table 6.1: Metabolic and Long-Term Health Effects of Elevated Cortisol Levels

Metabolic effect (cortisol-induced)	Chronic health condition
Increased appetite, accelerated muscle catabolism (breakdown), suppressed fat oxidation, enhanced fat storage	Obesity
Elevated cholesterol and triglyceride levels	Heart disease
Elevated blood pressure	Heart disease
Alterations in brain neurochemistry (involving dopamine and serotonin)	Depression/anxiety
Physical atrophy (shrinkage) of brain cells	Alzheimer's disease
Insulin resistance and elevated blood-sugar levels	Diabetes
Accelerated bone resorption (breakdown)	Osteoporosis
Reduced levels of testosterone and estrogen	Suppressed libido (reduced sex drive)
Suppression of immune-cell number and activity	Frequent colds/flu/infection
Reduced synthesis of brain neurotransmitters	Memory/concentration problems

followed by reduced sex-hormone levels and depressed libido (sex drive). That same year, a report from the New York Academy of Sciences suggested that elevated cortisol levels, caused by exposure to perceived stress, were associated with development of the metabolic syndrome (a.k.a. syndrome X) described in earlier chapters, which is characterized by insulin resistance, diabetes, abdominal obesity, elevated cholesterol, and hypertension. Research published in 2000 by scientists at Yale University supports the idea that emotional stress contributes to weight gain in both overweight and lean women. The researchers noted that the connection between stress and obesity is most likely due to an excessive secretion of cortisol and the adverse metabolic effects of the hormone in people with chronically elevated levels.

Elevated cortisol levels are also associated with reduced levels of testosterone and IGF-1 in men exposed to high stress. (IGF-1, or insulin-like growth factor 1, is a hormone related to growth hormone.) Because both testosterone and IGF-1 are anabolic or muscle-building hormones, these men also tend to have reduced muscle mass and higher body-fat levels. These same men also tend to have a higher body mass index (BMI), a higher waist-to-hip ratio (WHR), and abdominal obesity (an apple shape). Researchers at the Neurological Institute at the University of California at San Francisco (UCSF) have linked excessive cortisol levels to depression, anxiety, and Alzheimer's disease, as well as to direct changes in brain structure (atrophy) leading to cognitive defects (meaning that cortisol can shrink and kill brain cells).

So, as emphasized throughout this book, cortisol is not all bad—but too much of it for too long is a recipe for disaster. The sections that follow will outline in greater detail the metabolic relationship between elevated cortisol and specific conditions. Be warned: The news is not good for those of us who experience stress on a regular basis; the next section may even leave you feeling as if your high stress levels are killing you (and they are!). There is good news, however, and it starts in Chapter 7, where we'll begin to learn about the various steps that can help us get a handle on our stress response and help us modulate cortisol levels within a more healthful range.

HOW STRESS MAKES US FAT: CORTISOL, DIABETES, AND OBESITY

A primary focal point of this book is the close (and increasingly understood and acknowledged) relationship between stress, cortisol, and being overweight or obese. A key intermediary in the relationship (besides the aforementioned HSD enzyme and the hormone testosterone) is another hormone called *insulin*. Most people associate insulin problems with diabetes because of its primary role in regulating blood-sugar levels (although insulin has many additional functions in the body). Not only does insulin regulate blood-sugar levels within an extremely narrow range; it is also responsible for getting fat stored in our fat cells (adipose tissue), getting sugar stored in our liver and muscle cells (as glycogen), and getting amino acids directed toward protein synthesis (muscle building). Due to these varied actions, insulin is sometimes thought of as a "storage" hormone because it helps the body put all these great sources of energy away in their respective places for use later. That's great, but it is exactly the opposite of what the body experiences during the stress response, when the heart and muscles need lots of energy and need it fast.

One of the first signals the body must send out (via cortisol) during periods of stress is a message that screams, "No more energy storage!"—and that means shutting off the responsiveness of cells to the storage effects of insulin. When cells stop responding to insulin, they are able to switch from a storage (anabolic/building) mode to a secretion (catabolic/breakdown) mode—so fat cells dump more fat into the system, liver cells crank out more glucose, and muscle cells allow their protein to be broken down to supply amino acids (for conversion into even more sugar by the liver). This is all fine—assuming it occurs infrequently and for only a short period of time. Telling the body's cells to ignore insulin on a regular basis, as happens with chronic stress, can lead to a condition known as *insulin resistance* and predispose a person to the development of full-blown diabetes.

Stress makes a person fat primarily because of an excessive secretion of the key stress hormone, cortisol, along with a reduced secretion of key anabolic hormones, such as DHEA, testosterone, and growth hormone. This combination of highly catabolic cortisol and reduced anabolic hormones causes the body to store fat, lose muscle, slow metabolic rate, and increase appetite—all of which have the ultimate effect of making a person fatter. Overall, stress makes you burn fewer calories and consume more food (especially carbohydrates), which increases your stress levels even more! Even the *thought* of food and the *concern* about eating can increase stress levels—and therefore cortisol—in people who have restrained their eating habits and are either dieting or are concerned about their weight.

Scientific studies have shown that chronic stress clearly leads to overeating, which then leads to fat accumulation, frequently in the abdominal area. When we look at the relationship between stress and appetite, the picture can become a bit confusing—but it clears up when we look at the timing of the stress response. In the very early stages of stress, one hormone is secreted that *suppresses* appetite, while later in the stress response, another hormone is secreted to *increase* appetite. You'll remember from earlier chapters that, in response to stress, the hypothalamus in the brain gets the stress engines going by secreting CRH (corticotropin-releasing hormone). CRH kills the appetite. Now, before you get all excited and run off to order a month's supply of CRH over the Internet, you should also realize that although having more CRH available would certainly cut your appetite, it would also make you feel like you were having an anxiety or panic attack (not good).

Okay, so CRH *kills* appetite for the first few seconds of the stress response, but hot on its heels comes a dramatic rise in cortisol—which *stimulates* appetite (often by a lot) in the minutes to hours following the stressful event. CRH levels drop back to normal in seconds, while cortisol levels may take many hours to normalize—meaning that your appetite stays ramped up for a very long time (which drives you crazy until you finally succumb and eat something). Thought of in evolutionary terms, cortisol is actually quite a useful little hormone to have around; without it, our appetite would stay suppressed following a stressful event (such as running from the lion) and we'd never have the drive to refuel our depleted body. The obvious downside, of course, is that we're rarely expending huge amounts of energy when dealing with our modern stressors (sitting in a traffic jam doesn't burn very many calories), so the stimulated appetite makes us eat when we really don't need the calories—and we get fat.

Researchers have noticed that this pattern of accumulating abdominal fat during periods of stress is quite similar to a disease known as *Cushing's syndrome,* which is characterized by extremely high cortisol levels. In people afflicted with Cushing's syndrome, a prolonged exposure to excessive amounts of cortisol leads to massive accumulations of abdominal fat accompanied by severe loss of muscle tissue in the extremities (arms and legs). Many scientists now understand that the excessive cortisol production and tissue breakdown of Cushing's syndrome is similar in many ways to chronic cortisol exposure caused by repeated periods of stress (which can also lead to loss of vital bone and muscle tissue).

During periods of chronic stress, levels of both cortisol and insulin rise and together send a potent signal to fat cells to store as much fat as possible. They also signal fat cells to hold on to their fat stores—so stress can actually reduce the ability of the body to release fat from its stores to use for energy. In terms of weight gain and obesity, the link between cortisol and deranged metabolism is seen in many ways. These are listed in the sidebar below.

Metabolic Effects of Elevated Cortisol (Related to Weight Gain)

Loss of Muscle Mass

- Breakdown of muscles, tendons, and ligaments (to provide amino acids for conversion into glucose)
- Decreased synthesis of protein (to conserve amino acids for conversion into glucose)
- Reduced levels of DHEA, testosterone, growth hormone, IGF-1, and thyroid-stimulating hormone (TSH)
- Drop in basal metabolic rate (i.e., a reduced number of calories is burned throughout the day and night)

Increase in Blood-Sugar Levels

- Reduced transport of glucose into cells
- Decreased insulin sensitivity
- Increase in appetite and carbohydrate cravings

(cont'd.)

Increase in Body Fat
- Increase in the overall amount of body fat (due to increased appetite, overeating, and reduced metabolic rate)
- An accumulation of body fat in—and redistribution to—the abdominal region

From a vanity standpoint, nobody wants to carry around more body fat than they need to. From a health and longevity standpoint, elevated cortisol levels also tend to promote fat accumulation in the abdominal area, a condition that is closely associated with heart disease, diabetes, hypertension, and high cholesterol. Researchers are not completely sure why this "stress fat" accumulates specifically around the midsection. Its location here may have something to do with its being available for rapid access when the body needs additional fuel (because fat stored in the abdominal region can be delivered to the bloodstream and tissues faster then fat stored in peripheral regions such as the thighs and buttocks). But even though the *reason* for abdominal fat accumulation is still unclear, its *consequences* are well known. This combination of conditions, known as metabolic syndrome or syndrome X (as you may recall from earlier chapters), has been identified by many experts as the most important health danger that we'll face as a worldwide population in the early twenty-first century. (Syndrome X is covered in more detail in the next section.)

Most of us have grown fatter as we've grown older. It is interesting to note that several recent studies have demonstrated quite clearly that cortisol secretion increases and testosterone secretion decreases with aging, that elevated cortisol levels reduce our sensitivity to insulin, and that reduced insulin sensitivity is clearly linked to obesity, diabetes, and metabolic syndrome X. In some studies, overweight and obese subjects have been found to have cortisol levels in the normal range prior to meals, but within twenty to forty minutes after eating their cortisol levels surge. The effect of excessive cortisol secretion is also present for lean individuals, but overweight and obese people tend to exhibit the phenomenon to a much greater degree, leading several stress researchers to hypothesize that increased cortisol production may be one of the primary causative factors in weight gain.

There is certainly no shortage of observational studies showing the close relationship between hypercortisolemia (high blood levels of cortisol), hyperinsulinemia (high insulin levels), and reduced growth hormone (which in turn increases HSD activity). It is also interesting (and confusing) to note that some studies find no differences in the *absolute* cortisol levels between obese and lean subjects or between stressed and unstressed volunteers. What these studies *do* show, however, is an alteration in the normal secretory pattern of cortisol. This fluctuating pattern, when normal, should show the highest levels of cortisol in the morning, with a slow and gradual drop toward the lowest levels between midnight and 2:00 A.M. (refer back to Figure 3.2 on page 45).

Stressed-out subjects with an altered pattern of cortisol secretion are characterized by a low concentration of cortisol in the morning, the absence of a circadian rhythm, and a huge meal-related surge in cortisol levels (see Figure 6.1)—all of which are consistently associated with obesity and related measurements. People with disrupted

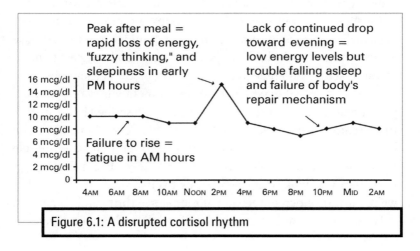

Figure 6.1: A disrupted cortisol rhythm

cortisol-secretion patterns have higher body fat (particularly in the abdomen), lower muscle mass (particularly in the arms and legs), and reduced basal metabolic rate (BMR, the number of calories burned at rest). On the other hand, the more "normal" pattern of cortisol metabolism (high in the morning, with a normal circadian rhythm) is associated with more favorable measures of body composition (more lean and less fat) as well as a healthier cardiovascular profile (lower blood pressure, reduced cholesterol and blood sugar, and better insulin sensitivity).

All in all, the above scenario makes for very discouraging news: Stress makes us fat. Even worse, however, may be the findings from researchers that have determined that the stress of *dieting* can make us fat. Why is this especially bad news? Primarily because at any given moment in our Western society, as much as 50 to 60 percent of the population is actively dieting—and many millions more are at least concerned about what they eat. This makes dieting one of the most common stress triggers, for both men and women—but why are so many people dieting? Aside from the obvious fact that few of us eat right or exercise enough, we also have to contend with mass-media messages equating thinness with beauty, success, and intelligence (and the implication that we can't achieve those things unless we are thin). Unfortunately, we also have to contend with the very real physiological changes that are occurring within each of us. As we age, our metabolic rate drops and most of us begin to pack on the pounds. Adding fat in the abdominal area (in response to stress) changes the body shape from that of an hourglass to more of a shot glass—and repeated diets only compound the problem.

Most of us will experience a drop in metabolism of about 0.5 percent per year after the age of twenty. (As described in Chapter 5, this situation is largely caused by a gradual decline in testosterone levels, which leads to a loss of about five to ten pounds of muscle tissue every decade.) Now, that may not seem like a large drop, but when you look at it over ten or twenty years, it means that we're burning 5 percent fewer calories at age thirty and 10 percent fewer calories at age forty—and so it goes, with about 5 percent fewer calories burned for every ten years of age (see Table 6.2). Just imagine: By the time we turn fifty, we're burning 15 percent fewer calories than we did when we were twenty. If you consume two thousand calories per day at age twenty (which is about average), this means you will need only seventeen hundred calories (three hundred fewer calories) at age fifty to maintain your body weight. It also means that if you don't make some serious changes in your diet and exercise patterns, or at least get your cortisol levels under control, then your fifty-year-old body will be carrying around over thirty extra pounds of fat than when you were twenty!

Table 6.2: Change in Metabolic Rate and Weight Gain with Age

Age (Years)	Daily Calorie Needs	Drop in Daily Metabolic Rate (from Age 20)	Pounds of Extra Fat (from Age 20)*
20	2,000–2,500		
30	1,900–2,375	100–125 calories	10
40	1,800–2,250	200–250 calories	20
50	1,700–2,125	300–375 calories	30
60	1,600–2,000	400–500 calories	40
70	1,500–1,875	500–625 calories	50

* without a corresponding change in diet/activity patterns

Remember that during periods of chronic stress, such as while dieting, rising cortisol levels send a potent signal to fat cells, telling them to store as much fat as possible. Cortisol also signals fat cells to hold on to their fat stores—so stress can actually reduce the ability of the body to release fat from its fat stores to use for energy. Does this mean that people with higher levels of stress are less able to lose weight? Yes, for a variety of reasons.

In one study, volunteers took part in a fifteen-week weight-loss program. They were put on a diet of seven hundred calories per day. As expected, the subjects experienced a significant increase in overall hunger, desire to eat, and total food consumption (when they were finally allowed to eat as much as they wanted). The most consistent predictor of these changes in desire to eat, fullness, and food intake was a change (an increase) in cortisol levels. The researchers hypothesized that the low-calorie diet induced a form of stress that increased cortisol levels and caused the people in the study to eat more—but it also may have simply been that the dieters were hungry because the researchers were starving them (after all, seven hundred calories per day is not a lot of food). So, to test the theory that the increase in hunger was caused by the stress/cortisol relationship rather than just by the severe diet, another study exposed a group of women to both a "stress session" and a "non-stress" (control) session on different days. The women who reacted to the stress by secreting higher levels of cortisol were the very same women who consumed more calories on the stress day compared to the low-stress day. Also of note was the fact that the women producing the most cortisol were not only hungrier, but they also showed an increase in negative moods in response to the stressors (which were significantly related to food consumption). These results suggest that stress itself, or at least the psychophysiological response to stress, can strongly influence cortisol levels and eating behavior, which, over time, could obviously have an impact on both weight and long-term health.

Okay, so now we know that the "stress" of a severe diet will make you hungry and cause you to eat more (regardless of the diet's calorie level). We also know that the stress without the diet will cause the very same thing to happen—but does this mean that *all* forms of stress will cause us to pork out? Maybe. Another study looked at a group of middle-aged men of varying socioeconomic grades (some were rich and some were poor). The fellows on the lower end of the socioeconomic ladder (the guys with less money) were significantly more likely to be overweight (visceral obesity) and to have higher cortisol values in relation to perceived stress (even though total cortisol secretion over the day of the study was not elevated). The researchers noted that the "duration of low socioeconomic conditions" (which is scientific mumbo jumbo for "being poor for a long time") seemed to worsen the effects of cortisol and strengthen the relationship between cortisol and obesity (meaning that being poor is bad for both your stress level and your waistline). Overall, the researchers concluded that the stress of a low socioeconomic status is associated with elevated cortisol secretion and also has a significant, strong, and consistent relationship with obesity. Closely related to pure socioeconomic studies of stress are the growing arguments that people eat more Big Macs, drink more Coke, and scarf more Oreos *not* because these companies tell us to eat them (via advertising), but because of stress. Lower socioeconomic populations may eat more junk food because they are more stressed out, not necessarily because Ronald McDonald invites them to "drive thru." Biology trumps advertising.

Perhaps one of the most compelling findings about the relationship between stress, cortisol, and obesity, however, comes from a study of young women by researchers at Yale University. Among these women, half of them had a high level of "cognitive dietary restraint," meaning they put a lot of mental energy into restricting themselves from overeating and/or from certain foods. Compared to women with low levels of cognitive dietary restraint, those with high restraint scores had significantly higher cortisol levels, despite also getting more exercise (in general, moderate levels of exercise tend to reduce stress and cortisol levels). Not only have the Yale scientists shown that high levels of stress can increase cortisol levels, but they have also been at the forefront in linking those high cortisol levels to accumulation of abdominal body fat (in both men and women) and to an accelerated loss of bone mass in young and old women (more on this later).

A number of similar studies conducted by the Department of Neurosciences at the New Jersey Medical School used rats to investigate the relationship between stress and obesity. Results from the animal studies showed that even moderate levels of daily, unpredictable stress over the course of five weeks led to increased levels of cortisol, increased appetite and food intake, and higher body weights compared to unstressed animals. The stressed-out rats had cortisol levels that were 48 percent higher than the mellow rats, and they ate 27 percent more and became 26 percent fatter. But what does that mean for us humans? Are we destined to become fat as a result of our stressful lives? Probably—unless we learn to control the adverse effects of cortisol.

Exercise and proper nutrition can certainly minimize our age-related drop in metabolism and increased tendency toward weight gain, but they can also help us control our response to stress and our metabolism of cortisol. The "right" program of diet and exercise will burn calories, shed fat, relieve stress, and reduce cortisol—but most people have enough experience with these "right" programs to know that diet and exercise have their own limitations. In fact, researchers at the University of Colorado have shown that athletes performing *too much* exercise (overtrained cross-country skiers) experience the very same adverse effects of elevated cortisol levels, such as mood disturbances, immune-system suppression, and increased levels of body fat. Of particular interest in this study was the finding that the athletes who were working out the most—those putting in the highest mileage and the longest training times—were also the ones with the highest cortisol levels, the highest body fat levels, and the poorest scores on measures of emotional outlook (more depression). Basically, they were exercising their brains out to get in better shape, but their elevated cortisol levels were hampering, and indeed outright *preventing,* their progress.

We have known for decades that dieting to lose weight is associated with significant muscle loss and impaired psychological function. Researchers from the Neurosciences Research Institute, in Birmingham, England, have recently shown that these effects are largely due to cortisol overexposure from "dieting stress," with "do-it-yourself" dieters showing a significant rise in cortisol levels after as little as one week of dieting.

Researchers from the University of Pittsburgh have suggested that a "chronic defeat response" may be at the root cause of certain cases of abdominal obesity and prediabetes. The hallmarks of chronic defeat include a high level of perceived stress and a greater tendency to mentally disengage from a stressful experience, both of which seem to lead to elevated cortisol exposure. It has been hypothesized that the repeated cycles of weight loss/regain that many Americans undergo is one form of a chronic defeat response, with repeat dieters increasing their risk of weight regain with each subsequent attempt.

Japanese nutrition researchers have shown that acute early-stage stress reduces appetite and food intake due to increased levels of corticotrophin-releasing hormone (CRH), but that during recovery from stress and during longer-term chronic stress, appetite becomes stimulated due to the effects of residual cortisol (which, as we've discussed, tends to persist in the systems of chronically stressed individuals).

In perhaps the most compelling argument for the impact of stress and cortisol in the epidemic of obesity in industrialized nations around the world, neuroscientist Mary Dallman and fellow scientists at the University of California at San Francisco have documented the dramatic effects of cortisol on food intake, metabolism, and abdominal obesity, and the profound effects of stress in our fast-paced modern societies globally.

So where does this leave us? In terms of weight loss, we know quite clearly that stress, dieting, and cortisol are all detrimental to our overall goals of shedding excess body fat. We also know from decades of research that both exercise and good nutrition can be helpful in controlling stress, cortisol, body weight, and a whole host of related health parameters. Scientists at the University of Göteborg, in Sweden, have shown that high cortisol levels are associated with a high waist-to-hip ratio, excess abdominal fat, elevated insulin levels, and a reduced secretion of growth hormone and testosterone—but they have also shown that a 13–14 percent reduction in cortisol levels is associated with a weight loss of more than twelve pounds. This means that despite the gloom and doom caused by the link between stress, cortisol, and obesity, we have some hope that by controlling cortisol levels we can make a positive impact on our body weight and level of body fat. Indeed, researchers from the University of Montreal have linked obesity to stress (higher stress levels = higher body weight), but have also found that education and mental outlook can reduce that stress/weight relationship. In a study across eleven worksites, individuals with higher levels of education and higher levels of optimism were less likely to gain weight in response to high stress levels. The "antistress" and weight-loss effects of education and mental outlook suggest that we *can* control the detrimental effects of cortisol overexposure—just as my research group has shown in numerous iterations of the SENSE Lifestyle Program over the last five years in our Utah nutrition clinic.

CORTISOL AND SYNDROME X

Most people have never even heard of syndrome X (also termed metabolic syndrome), which refers to a cluster of related conditions and symptoms including diabetes, insulin resistance, obesity, hypertension, high cholesterol, and heart disease (yikes!). If you are starting to gain weight, feeling low on energy, seeing your cholesterol level and blood pressure creep up, and feeling as if your mind is not quite as sharp as it used to be, you are a likely candidate for developing (or you are already suffering from) syndrome X.

One of the key metabolic aspects of syndrome X is insulin resistance (discussed in the previous section as it relates to obesity). Insulin resistance leads to a reduction in the body's cellular response to insulin, which interferes with blood-sugar regulation, increases appetite, and blocks the body's ability to burn fat. When insulin resistance is combined with a poor diet (high in fat and/or refined carbohydrates), the result is the metabolic syndrome known as syndrome X, which can have an impact on virtually every disease-inducing process in the body.

Some authors have proposed that both insulin resistance itself and syndrome X are *caused* by a diet high in refined carbohydrates such as cookies, soda, pasta, cereals, muffins, breads, rolls, and the like. While it is indeed true that refined carbohydrates (also known as *high-glycemic-index* carbohydrates) can raise blood levels of glucose and insulin, it is highly speculative that these junk foods actually *cause* syndrome X. (There's no controversy, however, that a diet high in such foods will certainly not help your health.) Instead, it is far more likely that the metabolic cascade of events set in motion by stress and elevated cortisol levels is the primary factor in getting a person started toward developing full-blown syndrome X—and a poor diet may hasten the trip.

People at highest risk for syndrome X are typically those of us who are approaching "middle age" (which is always a relative term). Aside from the fact that syndrome X simply leaves you feeling kind of "blah" (fatigued, fuzzy-headed, depressed, and disinterested in sex), it also sets the stage for several life-threatening conditions including obesity, heart disease, diabetes, Alzheimer's disease, and some forms of cancer.

Among the early signs of syndrome X are low energy levels and "fuzzy" mental functioning. Very often, these feelings strike following meals, due to the body's difficulty handling carbohydrates. A syndrome X sufferer will also notice that his clothes begin to fit a bit tighter due to a gradual weight gain of a pound or so at a time. Most problematically, the person will also have trouble *losing* those extra few pounds due to a variety of metabolic changes such as elevated blood sugar, increased insulin levels, and reduced levels of certain anabolic hormones (all of which you remember from the previous section about how stress makes us fat).

Taken separately, each of these relatively mild changes in one's metabolic machinery is not a big deal and is likely to be brushed off by the sufferer or his health-care provider with an overly simplistic recommendation to "get more exercise" or "watch what you eat." When considered *together*, however, the additive effect of each of these metabolic changes compounds a person's overall risk of serious health problems.

The primary effects of stress in raising one's risk of diabetes (only one aspect of syndrome X) are related to chronically elevated levels of glucose and insulin in the blood. Over time, elevated glucose and insulin cause the body's cells (primarily the ones in fat and muscle tissue) to become less sensitive to the effects of insulin, a condition known as *insulin resistance*. In response to the development of insulin resistance in these cells, the body begins to produce even more insulin—starting the vicious cycle that leads to development of full-blown diabetes.

Insulin resistance is perhaps one of the earliest metabolic events leading to full-blown syndrome X—and insulin resistance is certainly *exacerbated* by, if not exactly *caused* by, a diet high in refined carbohydrates (sugars) and by elevated cortisol levels (from chronic stress). Refined carbohydrates increase glucose and insulin levels in the blood, while cortisol reduces the effectiveness of insulin and reduces the body's ability to burn fat for energy. Both diet and exercise can play important roles in helping to control blood-sugar and insulin levels, but unless you adequately control cortisol levels, your attention to diet and exercise will leave you spinning your wheels.

Adding to the complexity of the connection between stress, cortisol, and metabolic alterations (e.g., insulin resistance), is the recent finding that inadequate sleep may actually contribute significantly to insulin resistance. This is particularly interesting because of the well-known link between sleep deprivation and elevated cortisol levels. In 2001, at the Annual Scientific Meeting of the American Diabetes Association, sleep researchers from the University of Chicago presented new evidence that inadequate sleep may promote the development of insulin resistance. The research team compared "normal" sleepers (averaging 7.5 to 8.5 hours of sleep per night) to "short" sleepers (averaging less than 6.5 hours of sleep per night), finding that the short sleepers secreted 50 percent more insulin and were 40 percent less sensitive to the effects of insulin compared to the normal sleepers. This is precisely the same effect seen during the aging process, when we begin to sleep fewer hours per night, our cortisol levels begin to rise, and our cells begin to become resistant to the effects of insulin.

Could inadequate amounts of sleep also be contributing to premature aging? Probably. The Chicago sleep researchers also suggested that sleep deprivation, which is becoming commonplace in industrialized countries, may play a significant role in the current epidemic of obesity and type-2 diabetes. A recent poll conducted by the National Sleep Foundation documents a steady decline in the number of hours Americans sleep each night. In 1910, the average American slept a whopping nine hours per night; in 1975, it was down to only about seven and a half hours; and today we average only about seven hours a night—and many of us get far less than that.

CORTISOL, FATIGUE, AND INSOMNIA

Mark was a building contractor who liked his job and enjoyed spending time with his family and on his hobbies (snowmobiling in winter and boating in summer). Because of his laid-back attitude, he appeared to be about as low-stress a person as you could ever meet. Unfortunately, he often reported problems with his sleep patterns; most notably, he had great difficulty falling asleep because his mind got going "a million miles an hour" as soon as he retired for the evening. Mark would often wake up in the middle of the night and have trouble dropping off again. The lack of sleep was beginning to affect his work. First of all, he had a hard time getting out of bed on time in the mornings, and then once he was at work he had trouble concentrating on the precise measurements and craftsmanship necessary to do his job. How did Mark finally deal with his stress-induced insomnia and fatigue? To find out, see Chapter 8.

How do you suppose it is that stress can cause us to be fatigued during the day—but also cause us to have trouble falling asleep at night? The "dynamic duo" of chronic fatigue and insomnia would logically seem to be opposite conditions (if you're so tired, why can't you fall asleep?), but they are commonly found together in the two-thirds of the American population who report experiencing chronic stress and who get inadequate sleep. The common element? You guessed it: cortisol. Making matters worse is the fact that insomnia and fatigue often combine with each other in a vicious cycle wherein stress makes it hard to relax and fall asleep, a person's fatigued condition the next day makes stressors harder to deal with, and the additional stress causes even more difficulty falling asleep the next night (see Figure 6.2).

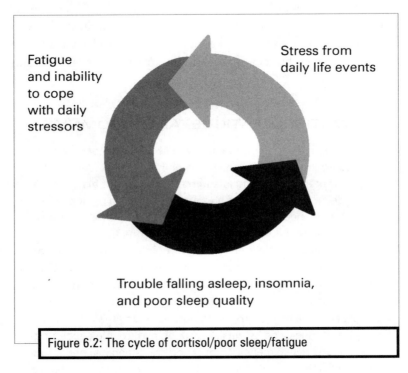

Fatigue and inability to cope with daily stressors

Stress from daily life events

Trouble falling asleep, insomnia, and poor sleep quality

Figure 6.2: The cycle of cortisol/poor sleep/fatigue

But how, exactly, does cortisol fit into this picture? As we all know by now, cortisol levels are elevated in response to stress, so any stressful events encountered in the late afternoon to early evening will hamper a person's ability to relax and fall asleep that night. If you'll recall, one of the many effects of cortisol is to increase a person's level of alertness—which is exactly what you want to avoid right before bedtime. Also, if you don't get to bed at a reasonable hour (early enough to allow a full eight to nine hours of shut-eye), your cortisol metabolism doesn't get a chance to follow its normal rhythm, which would achieve its lowest point around 2:00 A.M., as illustrated earlier. As a result, you may get only five, six, or seven hours of sleep, and you wake up groggy after having been exposed to higher than normal levels of cortisol throughout the night.

The long-term results of sleeping less than the standard eight hours a night are annoying side effects such as headaches, irritability, frequent infections, depression, anxiety, confusion, and generalized mental and physical fatigue. But it's not just that a lack of sleep leaves you feeling crappy; research shows that even mild sleep deprivation can actually destroy one's long-term health and increase one's risk of diabetes, obesity, and breast cancer. In many ways, sleeping less than eight hours each night is as bad for overall wellness as gorging on junk food or becoming a couch potato.

Remember that cortisol levels normally peak in the early morning (about 6:00 A.M. to 8:00 A.M.) as a way to get a person moving and prepare her to face the challenges of the day. Between 8:00 A.M. and 11:00 A.M., cortisol levels begin to drop, and they continue to gradually decline throughout the day, typically causing us to feel a decrease in energy levels and ability to concentrate sometime around 3:00 P.M. to 4:00 P.M. (the "afternoon slump"). This dip in energy levels is the body's way of saying, "The day is almost over; better get ready for sleep." Unfortunately, instead of getting ready for sleep, our modern lifestyles cause most of us to search for a way to boost our energy levels in the evenings so that we can get through soccer practices, piano recitals, business dinners, and time with our families. Our body clock really wants us to eat our last meal of the day around 5:00 P.M. and to be asleep by 8:00 P.M., but our wristwatch has us awake late into the night. The major problem with our modern "late to bed, early to rise" lifestyles is that our cortisol levels never have enough time to fully dissipate (which is supposed to happen overnight), so our bodies never have a chance to fully recover and repair themselves from the detrimental effects of chronic stress.

The natural rhythm of *restful* sleep follows a very specific path from the moment your head hits the pillow: breathing slows, muscles relax, heart rate and blood pressure drop, and body temperature falls. The brain releases melatonin (the "sleep hormone") and begins its change from the rapid beta waves (indicating daytime restless wakefulness) to the slower alpha waves (indicating calm wakefulness) and eventually to the still slower theta waves that predominate during the various stages of sleep. During a full night of sleep, we normally pass through several stages of sleep: Stage 2 (lasting ten to fifteen minutes), then Stage 3 (lasting five to fifteen minutes), and finally to the deepest portion of sleep in Stage 4 (lasting about thirty minutes), and the most famous portion of the sleep cycle, REM (rapid eye movement), when we dream. This cycle, from Stage 2 to REM sleep, takes an average of ninety minutes to complete and will repeat itself over and over throughout the night. In the absence of alarm clocks, lights, and other interruptions, sleep researchers have found that the natural duration of these repeating sleep cycles (the "physiological ideal") is eight hours and fifteen minutes.

So what happens to those of us who simply can't (or won't) get that much shut-eye? Well, for one thing, blood-sugar levels will rise. Sleep researchers have shown that getting only four hours of sleep per night results in signs of impaired glucose tolerance and insulin resistance—which means that as little as a few nights of cheating on sleep can put a person in a prediabetic state. These changes in insulin action and blood-sugar control are also linked to the development of obesity. Compounding the link between obesity and poor sleep is the fact that levels of both growth hormone and leptin are reduced in people who spend less time in deep sleep. (Leptin is a hormone with important roles in regulating appetite, body weight, metabolism, and reproductive function.) Less growth hormone in the system typically means a loss of muscle and a gain of fat over time, while reduced levels of leptin will lead to hunger and carbohydrate cravings.

Let's look at the case of a typical all-American go-getter; we'll call him Driven Dan. Who's got time for sleep? Dan can't worry about the abstract risks of getting fat, developing diabetes, or con-tracting cancer—he has work to do, classes to take, bills to pay, soccer practices to attend, yada, yada, yada. Sound familiar? So what's the solution? Perish the thought that our friend Dan should try to do fewer things—you'll get none of that "simplify your life" stuff in this book (despite the fact that it makes perfect sense). In an ideal world, Dan may be able to work seven hours a day, enjoy a short commute to work, and have all the free time he can stand. In the real world, however (the one in which we all live), the more realistic approach for Dan (and for you?) may be to do the next best thing by getting a handle on his cortisol levels, a topic we'll delve into in the next few chapters.

CORTISOL AND SEX DRIVE

Holly and *Alan* were happily married young newlyweds with a big problem. As newlyweds, one of the things that should have held great interest for them (SEX!) offered little allure. The prob-lem was certainly not their love and attraction for each other, but their extreme stress levels. Both Holly and Alan were (and still are) ambitious young professionals, with long stressful hours at the office and all the trappings of financial success; both had MBAs, drove BMWs, and lived in a beautiful home paid for by two sizable incomes. The good news is that Holly and Alan were able to reignite the spark in their love life. Learn how they did so in Chapter 8.

You don't need to read a book about the relationship between stress and disease to know that when we're stressed out we also have problems in the "intimacy" department. For starters, menstrual cy-cles get all out of whack, erections are more difficult to achieve and maintain, and overall libido (sex drive) plummets. Stress simply makes us lose interest in sex. In males, this is due primarily to a dra-matic fall in testosterone levels during stressful times. In females, the stress-induced loss of sex drive is a bit more complicated, in-volving disruption in levels not only of testosterone, but also of estrogen, progesterone, and prolactin.

The stress/libido relationship is, predictably, tied to cortisol levels (and also to another class of chemicals from the brain—the endorphins—but more on them later). In men, elevated cortisol levels do at least a few things to suppress our sex drive. First, cortisol signals the body to reduce its production of the "prehormone" compounds that serve as the precursors to testosterone. Cut off the supply of "parts" and your production of the end product also dries up. Next, just in case any testosterone *does* get produced, cortisol also blocks the normal response of the testicles to testosterone, which is generally to make guys feel frisky. This also means that supplemental forms of testosterone, such as anabolic steroids and dietary supplements that contain DHEA or androstenedione, are less likely to have any effects on libido when you're under stress. Finally, if we think for a moment about the actual mechanics of achieving an erection, it is obvious that we need a redistribution of blood flow from one place to another. When you're under stress, however, blood is being channeled to places where it can provide the most benefit, like your arms for fighting or your legs for fleeing, not to your privates.

Let's get back to the endorphins. These are the "feel-good," pain-relieving chemicals released by the brain, and they are responsible for the euphoric feeling known as "runner's high." The interesting thing about endorphins is that they also work to suppress some of the hormonal steps leading to testosterone production. This helps to explain the findings from studies of extreme endurance athletes wherein high levels of endorphins and cortisol are associated with low testosterone levels, reduced sperm counts, and reduced sex drive. This is not to say that aerobic exercise, such as jogging or cycling, is *bad* for you, but it emphasizes the fact that *extremes* of exercise (and inadequate recovery) are perceived by the body as stressors—and, in reaction, the body goes through the same stress response caused by other stressful events.

In women, the relationship between stress and sexual/reproductive function is a bit more complicated. In very basic terms, the menstrual cycle can be divided into two distinct phases. In the first phase, known as the *follicular phase,* estrogen is the dominant hormone (although there are several important hormones interacting here) and ovulation (the release of an egg from the ovaries) is the primary event. The second phase of the menstrual cycle, known as the *luteal phase,* is dominated by an increase in another hormone, progesterone, which stimulates the uterus to get ready for implantation of a fertilized egg (assuming that the newly released egg meets up with an eligible sperm). Failing fertilization, the thickened uterine lining is lost in the form of blood and tissue during menstruation, and the whole cycle repeats itself in another twenty-eight days (give or take a couple days).

During stress, this extremely complex and tightly regulated hormonal balance gets all out of whack. Estrogen and progesterone levels drop (so eggs are not released from the ovaries, a condition called *anovulation*), and the uterine lining remains undeveloped (so eggs cannot be implanted). Menstrual cycles can become irregular (oligomenorrhea) or cease altogether (amenorrhea). Speaking of amenorrhea, it is interesting to note that female athletes often encounter disruptions in their menstrual cycles as a result of their training and eating patterns. Just as with the male endurance athletes (and their low testosterone levels) mentioned above, these female athletes tend to have low levels of estrogen and progesterone as well as a severely reduced libido. They also tend to be dieting or at least not consuming enough calories to support the energy demands of their sport. If you think about it, the fact that they have no interest in sex (or the ability to get pregnant) makes perfect sense. The change in hormone levels and the demands of their diet and exercise regimens are being perceived by the body as major stressors. Because the average pregnancy burns up about fifty thousand calories (and afterward another thousand calories per day for breast-feeding), it is quite logical for the body to shut off its sexual desire (and ability) during stressful times.

So what to do? Quit your job, move to the islands, and open a surf shop! Your sex drive is *guaranteed* to increase. (Ever wonder why you feel friskier when you're on vacation? Less stress!) Not practical to move your family to Tahiti? Okay, but then at least do something about your cortisol levels. Solutions are presented in upcoming chapters.

CORTISOL, SUPPRESSED IMMUNE FUNCTION, AND CANCER

We know that during periods of increased stress, there is also often an increase in the incidence of certain chronic conditions such as asthma, allergies, and rheumatoid arthritis, as well as of gastrointestinal ailments such as irritable bowel syndrome (IBS) and Crohn's disease. This is quite interesting, because each of these conditions is considered to have an autoimmune component to it—meaning that one's own immune system has gone a bit haywire and has started to attack one's own tissues. In these cases, doctors often prescribe synthetic versions of cortisol as a way to suppress an overactive immune system, and it works quite well—but only for a short period of time. The problem with using synthetic cortisol as a medication, however, is that too much of the stuff, or even a modest amount for too long, leads to the very same tissue breakdown and metabolic disturbances that occur when experiencing chronic stress.

Medical researchers have known for more than sixty years that chronic or repeated bouts of stress will lead to a shrinking of the thymus gland (one of the key immune tissues in the body) and to a general suppression of immune-system strength. We know that cortisol has a direct effect on shrinking the thymus and inhibiting white blood cell production and activity. Cortisol suppresses the ability of white blood cells to secrete chemical messengers (interleukins and interferons), so the different varieties of immune-system cells become unable to communicate with each other in a way that would allow them to more effectively fight off infections. Finally, and most remarkably, is the fact that cortisol can actually act as a signal to many immune-system cells to simply shut off and stop working (that is, the cells die).

Now, why would stress and cortisol have all of these detrimental effects on the immune system? You would think that during times of stress, the body would want to *increase* its resistance to invading pathogens (bacteria and viruses) rather than *decrease* this vital protection—but this is clearly not what happens. To answer this question we need to again consider the *timing* of the stress response. Just as the relationship between cortisol and appetite has an aspect of timing to it (stress suppresses appetite for a few seconds or minutes, but then stimulates appetite for the next few hours), the relationship between cortisol and immune-system function is also mediated by timing. If we look at stress/immunity in these terms, we see that immune function is actually *stimulated* by stress for a short period of time (a few minutes). This short blast of immune-system stimulation appears to be used by the body to "wake up" existing immune-system cells as well as to "clear out" cells that fail to work properly due to normal cell aging.

This is all very good: Now you have a short-term stressor that has ramped up immune-system activity and you're ready to fight off the invading bugs. The problem, as it has been for many of the bodily systems discussed thus far, is that a *prolonged* stress response sends these finely regulated systems into complete chaos. During periods of chronic stress, cortisol levels remain elevated and immune-system integrity begins to suffer. Not only do the chronically stimulated immune-system cells start to break down, losing their ability to fight off invading pathogens, but in some cases they can start to unleash their destructive properties on the body's own tissues, resulting in a variety of allergies, as well as in autoimmune diseases such as multiple sclerosis, lupus, fibromyalgia, and rheumatoid arthritis (see Figure 6.3 on the next page).

Confused yet? If not, then you should be, because most of the world's top immunologists and stress physiologists are baffled by the fact that stress increases immune-system function on the one hand, but then turns around and dismantles one of our most important protective systems on the other. One of the proposed reasons for

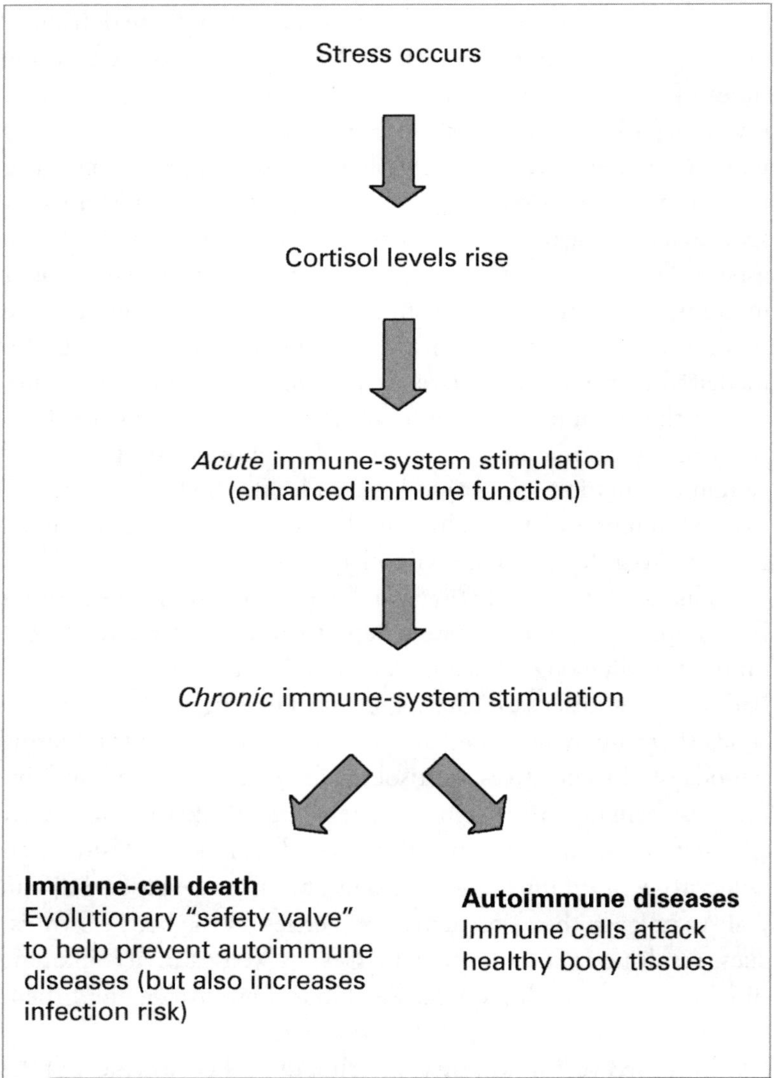

Stress occurs

Cortisol levels rise

Acute immune-system stimulation
(enhanced immune function)

Chronic immune-system stimulation

Immune-cell death
Evolutionary "safety valve"
to help prevent autoimmune
diseases (but also increases
infection risk)

Autoimmune diseases
Immune cells attack
healthy body tissues

Figure 6.3: The relationship between stress, cortisol, and immune
function

this "Jekyll and Hyde" effect of cortisol has to do with the fact that while a stimulated immune system is good on a short-term basis, undergoing this stimulation on a long-term basis may actually lead to autoimmune diseases (wherein the immune system attacks the body's own tissues).

It makes good sense for cortisol to stimulate immune-system activity during stress, and when cortisol levels return to normal (after the stress is over) for overall immune-system activity to normalize as well. Unfortunately, our modern high-stress lifestyles (the Type C condition) don't allow cortisol levels to return to normal. Consequently, one of the body's "safety valves" comes into play, whereby chronic exposure to cortisol causes the immune-system cells to break down, thus preventing autoimmune diseases, but also reducing our ability to ward off future infections and increasing our risk for many diseases.

Speaking of autoimmune diseases, it is important to make the point (again) that glucocorticoids (of which cortisol is one) are routinely used by physicians to combat autoimmune diseases. If we think of autoimmune diseases as conditions wherein an overactive immune system attacks our joints (rheumatoid arthritis) or nerve cells (multiple sclerosis) or connective tissue (lupus), then it is logical to knock down this overzealous immune system with a huge dose of cortisol (glucocorticoids). In this way, cortisol can be thought of as our "friend" by suppressing immune-system activity, but cortisol can also be thought of as our "enemy" because of the memory problems, muscle loss, and other side effects experienced by patients injected with high doses of glucocorticoids. Unfortunately, during times of stress these very same autoimmune diseases tend to flare up—which is confusing, because the stress-induced rise in cortisol would be expected to reduce immune-system activity and actually help control the diseases. Again, it probably comes down to timing, with short-term stress causing a temporary stimulation of immune activity and, thus, an increase in the symptoms of the autoimmune condition.

Studies in both animals and humans have noted a reduction by as much as 50 percent in levels of immune-system cells called *natural killer cells* following exposure to various forms of stress. Natural killer cells (NK cells) typically function within the immune system to identify viruses and cancer cells. In one study of breast cancer patients, the level of emotional stress caused by the initial cancer diagnosis was directly related to NK cell activity. In these women, a higher stress level predicted a reduced ability of NK cells to destroy cancer cells as well as a poorer response to interventions aimed at improving NK cell activity. From animal studies, we know that cortisol not only suppresses the number and activity of NK cells, but also promotes the synthesis of new blood vessels in tumors (a process called *angiogenesis*) and accelerates the growth of certain kinds of tumors. The bottom line here may be that chronic stress can accelerate the growth of cancer cells in the body as well as block the body's ability to battle the disease.

Heightened stress levels have also been linked to adverse effects on the balance of intestinal microflora, which are known to respond to changes in both diet and stress level. These beneficial bacteria live in our intestinal tract, and in addition to being intimately involved with optimal gastrointestinal function (more on this later), they also play a vital role in helping to support immune function. In a study of fighter pilots preparing for simulated battle (a fairly stressful event), distinct reductions were noted in the numbers of "good" bacteria (lactobacilli and bifidobacteria), along with a corresponding increase in the numbers of "bad" bacteria (*E. coli,* enterobacteria, and clostridia). The outcome for these pilots was, predictably, a sharp increase in their reported incidence of sore throats, headaches, colds, diarrhea, and upset stomachs.

Numerous studies in animals and humans have shown that both acute and chronic stress increases susceptibility to infectious diseases. In particular, the risk of developing upper-respiratory-tract infections (URTIs) is sharply increased, so that people who are under the greatest stress (or who deal with it poorly) are the ones who most often get these types of sicknesses. Students catch colds during exam week, and accountants get sore throats in April, when they're filing dozens of last-minute tax returns.

In some stress-management clinics, the primary ways to determine whether or not a given person will get sick include:

- The number of major life events in the past year (divorce, death in the family, change in job or location, etc.)
- A psychological perception that daily demands exceed coping resources and/or support system
- Their current emotional state

Researchers have found that the first of these three "sickness determinants," the overall degree of psychological stress, is strongly related, in a dose-response fashion, to URTIs (upper-respiratory-tract infections) and other breakdowns in immune-system integrity (such as gastrointestinal health). This means the more stressed out you are, the more likely you are to get sick.

Swedish researchers have found chronic stress to increase the occurrence of yeast infections, a consequence likely due to the overall suppression of immune-system activity caused by the stress. Brazilian researchers have linked elevated stress to both depression and suppressed immune function, and they have suggested that chronic stress may contribute to the development of certain forms of cancer. In a series of experiments, results show that various cellular and molecular aspects of the immune system are impaired in patients suffering from chronic stress and depression, yielding, for example, high levels of cortisol and inflammatory cytokines, and reduced numbers and activity of T cells and NK cells, the specific immune-cell types responsible for the immune system's surveillance of cancer tumors.

We have known for many years that some forms of cancer are related to increased levels of psychological stress. Researchers from the University of Wisconsin Medical School have recently shown that breast cancer patients who have a flattened cortisol rhythm (resulting in an elevated twenty-four-hour exposure to cortisol) are more likely to have a poor prognosis/outcome than their counterparts with normal cortisol rhythms.

So after all this discussion about the suppression of immune-system function due to stress, who do you think gets sick most often? What demographic group, among all others, suffers from the highest incidence of stress-related disease?

- Wealthy investment bankers? No.

- Stressed-out college students? No.

- Single mothers working two jobs and driving beat-up 1985 Ford Escorts? Yes!

The most direct example of the chronically elevated human stress response can be observed every day in the lives of a large part of the American (and worldwide) population. These are the folks who are driving a junker car (and hoping it makes it) to their second job. They are hoping the money from that second paycheck will last until the end of the month when the bills are due. They are *not* the people whom you see commiserating with each other about their terrible jobs on sitcoms such as *Friends*. The constant unrelenting stress of making ends meet, job instability, sleep deprivation, poor diet, lack of outlets for stress, and overall lack of control combine to increase the risk of disease by a factor of five to ten!

Unfortunately, none of the information or recommendations that follow in this book will alleviate the actual stressors encountered by the "working poor" or the "working middle class" (wherever you choose to draw the economic line)—but much of what follows can be used to reduce the damage wreaked by stress on all of us.

CORTISOL AND CARDIOVASCULAR DISEASE

A large and exceedingly important part of the stress response is its direct and rapid effect on the cardiovascular system. As outlined previously, the fight-or-flight response is meant to prepare your body for forceful physical activity. But no matter whether you're saved by your fists (fight) or your feet (flight), your cardiovascular system had better be ready to support whatever vigorous activity you decide to undertake. This means ramping up heart rate, blood pressure, and cardiac output (the amount of blood your heart pumps). It also means shutting down certain nonessential uses of blood, such as digestion, and shunting that blood to more important areas—like the arms and legs, where it can fuel the fighting/fleeing muscles. Shunting blood around the body means coordinating the dilation (relaxation) of some blood vessels and the constriction (narrowing) of others, an effect that results in elevated blood pressure during periods of stress.

What a great set of effects! If you were a race car, this stress-induced series of events would be analogous to a supercharger, and—ZOOM!—away you'd dash. The key problem may already be apparent to you: Keep that supercharger opened full throttle for too long, or use it too frequently, and you're likely to blow a gasket, throw a piston, or destroy the entire engine. What this means for your heart and cardiovascular system is clear: Chronic activation of your stress-response system increases your risk of blowing a gasket in your heart—otherwise known as heart disease.

We know that elevated blood pressure can accelerate damage to the interior lining of blood vessels. These small areas of vessel damage become perfect "docking points" for circulating particles of sugar, fat, and cholesterol—so there they stick (and stress has already elevated each of them to serve as fuel for your expected fight/flight). As if that weren't already bad enough, your blood gets thicker because stress hormones have a tendency to promote blood clotting. Thick blood might be a good thing if you come out on the losing side of a fight, but it's not a good thing if you're simply sitting in a traffic jam with a rapid heart rate, elevated blood pressure, and constricted blood vessels.

A variety of animal studies (in monkeys, rats, mice, and dogs) has supported the concept that stress leads to heart disease. Across these studies, it is clear that the animals subjected to the most *social* stress are also the ones that develop the most or worst blockages in their blood vessels. High-fat diets appear to compound the problems (duh!). Interestingly, *physical* stressors do not seem to be quite as bad for the heart, probably because running around, wrestling, or fighting appear to help dissipate stress hormones.

Health professionals have known for decades that blood pressure, cholesterol levels, heart attacks, and strokes are closely related to overall degree of stress. Emotional state has been known to trigger heart attacks in many people, with feelings of sadness, anger, and "control" (that is, how much or how little control people feel they have over their lives and/or destinies) being linked to causation of heart disease. Overall, risk for coronary heart disease is three to five times greater in people with higher levels of anger, anxiety, and worry compared to people who report lower levels.

Researchers from the Mayo Clinic have shown that psychological stress is one of the strongest risk factors for heart attacks. Furthermore, when calculating the economic costs of a high-stress lifestyle, economists have shown that hospital usage costs more than $9,500 per visit in heart-attack patients with high stress, but just over $2,100 in those with low stress.

Most of us understand that heart disease is the leading cause of death in the United States and much of the Western world. Almost all cases of heart attack and stroke are due to atherosclerosis caused by high blood pressure, high cholesterol, diabetes (high blood-sugar and insulin levels), smoking, and physical inactivity. What many people fail to realize, however, is that the cardiovascular aspects of heightened stress may merely be the tip of the iceberg when it comes to the long-term health consequences of elevated cortisol levels.

The good news is that there also appears to be a powerful inverse relationship between stress and the strength of one's social network—meaning that strong social support (from friends, family, and coworkers) can be a key factor in reducing the link between stress and heart disease. Stated another way, those with a stronger social network can withstand more stress before succumbing to disease. More good news is found in reports of the association between stress and hypertension: The dissipation of stress, through either meditation or exercise, helps to bring blood pressure back to normal levels.

YOUR BRAIN ON CORTISOL: ANXIETY, DEPRESSION, AND ALZHEIMER'S DISEASE

Rachel was a single mom with two young children. In addition to her full-time job at her daughter's day care, she also volunteered as a chaperone for her son's Boy Scout troop. As you can imagine, Rachel had more than enough stress in her life in the form of financial constraints, child-care issues, and being a single parent. As a result, she often felt her patience wearing thin, especially when confronted with a dozen screaming Boy Scouts at the end of a stressful day at the day care. Take a look at Chapter 8 to see how Rachel used specific nutritional supplements to deal with heightened anxiety and irritability.

Who among us is not affected to some degree by periods of stress and anxiety? For virtually everybody, modern lifestyles create a fair amount of tension, irritability, worry, and frustration, which can lead to feelings of chronic anxiety and depression. In fact, somewhere between 5 and 20 percent of Americans will experience depression severe enough to warrant medication or other therapy.

In addition to the emotional effects brought on by chronic stress are its direct effects on the brain. Research has shown that stress can increase the incidence of simple forgetfulness and accelerate the development of full-blown memory loss and Alzheimer's disease. Each of these conditions involves a degree of mental deterioration characterized by damage to and death of nerve cells in the brain—and it has been estimated that as many as 30 to 50 percent of adults in industrialized countries suffer from these conditions.

The changes in mood that accompany periods of heightened stress also bring reduced energy levels, feelings of fatigue, irritability, inability to concentrate, and feelings of depression—all of which are related to the same class of brain chemicals, the *neurotransmitters*. Most notable (and scary), perhaps, are the findings that chronic stress can lead to actual *physical* changes in the arrangement of the neurons (nerve cells) in the brain. In other words, we're talking now about stress changing both the function and the *shape* of your brain. No wonder it sometimes doesn't seem to work the way it's supposed to!

Related to depression, but different in a number of ways, is anxiety—that nagging, sometimes overwhelming, sense of disquiet or unease that most of us experience to one degree or another, at least occasionally. Anxiety can get completely out of hand if it takes the form of panic attacks or obsessive-compulsive disorder, both of which appear to be associated with a chronically overactive stress response (and especially with elevated catecholamines; that is, epinephrine and norepinephrine).

Panic disorder occurs in approximately 1 to 2 percent of the population. It typically begins in young adulthood, and women are twice as likely as men to suffer from it. The condition manifests itself in episodes of extreme anxiety and fear. These panic attacks, as they are commonly known, can last from a few seconds to a few hours and may include real physical symptoms such as shortness of breath, sweating, irregular heartbeat, dizziness, and faintness. They can be so severe that the sufferer ends up in the emergency room with fears that she or he is having a heart attack. Compounding the condition is the anticipatory anxiety that plagues the sufferer after experiencing these attacks, leading to a vicious cycle in which more anxiety is caused by worrying about having future panic attacks. It is unclear in these situations whether elevated cortisol levels are the primary causative factor that *induces* the panic attacks, or whether high cortisol levels *result from* the initial panic attack and, while remaining elevated, exacerbate the condition and set the stage for another attack.

Another variant of anxiety is obsessive-compulsive disorder (OCD), which produces obsessive, almost inescapable thoughts and compulsive behaviors the sufferer cannot help but perform. About 2 percent of the population suffers from OCD. Females are slightly more susceptible than males, and, as with panic disorder, it typically first manifests in young adulthood. People with OCD are in a sense better adapted to anxiety than are individuals with panic disorder, because those with OCD avoid panic attacks via their compulsive behaviors, which may act in a way as "de-stress" exercises. Unfortunately, the behaviors or rituals needed to satisfy the obsession/compulsion often interfere with normal activities and relationships. Most of the compulsions fall into one of four categories: checking, cleaning, counting, and avoidance. In many cases, it is thought that these compulsions act as simple defense mechanisms, whereby the compulsive behavior or obsessive thought patterns help to reduce feelings of anxiety. However, these thoughts and behaviors become ritualized and inescapable, leading to a heightened level of stress and anxiety as they begin to disrupt activities of daily living. Treatment for OCD generally involves both behavioral therapy and drug treatment, but the disorder often persists over time unless the root cause of the stress is fully addressed.

Clearly, various treatments exist for people suffering from anxiety. Aside from behavioral therapy, which is often all that is needed (especially for simple phobias), several medicinal treatments exist that vary according to the type of anxiety and whether or not the anxiety is combined with other problems. Traditional tranquilizers, such as Valium, are often the first medications that come to mind. However, anxiety frequently goes hand in hand with depression, and antidepressants such as Prozac, Zoloft, and Wellbutrin are often prescribed to treat the combination of problems. For individuals who prefer a more "natural" approach to treatment, there are many alternatives in the form of supplements, herbs, and combination products that may help alleviate anxiety, reduce stress, and control cortisol levels. These are covered in detail in upcoming chapters.

The ultimate cause of depression is exceedingly complex—and well beyond the scope of this book. From our perspective relating to the association of stress with depression, however, it is known that cortisol levels tend to be higher in people suffering from depression, while levels of brain neurotransmitters such as dopamine, norepinephrine, and serotonin are lower. Does this mean that cortisol lowers brain neurotransmitters or causes depression? Not necessarily, but we know quite clearly that the people who are under the highest levels of stress also tend to be the ones who succumb to periods of moderate depression. Part of the reason may be that during periods of heightened stress, the brain becomes accustomed to high cortisol levels, and when the stressor is removed (or reduced) the brain is unable to function effectively. We know from animal studies, for example, that the brains of rats exposed to repeated stresses eventually become resistant to specific pleasure pathways; therefore, higher and higher levels of the brain's "feel-good" chemicals (dopamine, serotonin, and endorphins) are needed to induce a response. It has also been known for more than twenty years that patients given high doses of cortisol-like drugs (such as corticosteroids to treat autoimmune diseases) also tend to develop memory problems and signs of clinical depression.

So, in asking ourselves the question "Does cortisol cause depression?," the answer is definitely, probably "maybe." It certainly appears that having elevated cortisol levels raises one's risk of developing depression. It also appears that cortisol does a pretty good job of gumming up the works when it comes to the synthesis, transport, breakdown, and overall activity of the neurotransmitters in the brain. Finally, we also know that using specialized drugs to "shut off" the production of cortisol can reduce the symptoms of depression—but these drugs, known as *adrenal steroidogenesis inhibitors*, have a list of nasty side effects as long as your arm.

Again, however, if we look at the relationship between stress and brain function, we see a two-phase effect, wherein short-term stress appears to enhance cognitive function, while chronic stress disrupts many aspects of brain neurochemistry. Researchers theorize that it works something like this: Acute stress causes an increase in blood flow, oxygen, and glucose to the muscles (for fight/

flight), and also to the brain. We know that hypoglycemia (low blood sugar) can impair concentration and ability to think, so the increased supply of glucose should, at least transiently, increase brainpower. And it does; studies of people exposed to short-term stressors show that they have an enhanced memory capacity and ability for problem solving. Unfortunately, the brain-boosting effects of stress are short-lived (lasting less than thirty minutes), because when the body is fully awash in cortisol, blood flow and glucose delivery to the brain begin to fall. Prolonged exposure of brain cells (neurons) to cortisol reduces their ability to take up glucose (their only fuel source) and—here's the really scary part—causes them to shrink in size! So there you have it. Repeated stress and prolonged exposure to cortisol—once again, the Type C condition—actually lead to a progressive destruction of the neurons in the brain. Not good.

The connection between adult-onset (type-2) diabetes and depression has been known since the late 1600s, when British physicians noted that diabetes was more common in people who suffered long-term sorrow. The link between stress/depression and diabetes/obesity (now often referred to as "diabesity") has also been known for many years, but it is just within the past decade or so that cortisol has emerged as the linchpin between the conditions. Cortisol builds up during depression, which could directly trigger a tendency toward "diabesity." Indeed, researchers from the University of Michigan have shown that reducing the conversion of inactive cortisol into active cortisol in fat cells (using flavonoids, as described in Chapter 4) results in a drop in cortisol levels of 45 to 73 percent and a reduction in abdominal fat of 10 to 13 percent within twelve weeks. Another group of Dutch researchers has found that being depressed increases a person's risk of developing diabetes by 37 percent—about equal to the risk posed by smoking or lack of exercise.

A group of researchers from the National Institute of Occupational Health, in Copenhagen, Denmark, have recently shown that "bullying" at work increases stress levels and is associated with adverse health outcomes. Workers who indicated having been bullied on the job reported more symptoms of depression, anxiety, and overall stress, accompanied by elevated cortisol levels. It was interesting to note in these studies that while daytime levels of cortisol were elevated in the bullied workers (indicating high stress levels at work), their "waking" cortisol levels were suppressed (indicating a high risk of developing stress disorders such as chronic fatigue and fibromyalgia). A similar series of studies by German researchers at the University of Trier found that higher measures of cortisol at work were associated with workers feeling more tense, angry, and unhappy.

Mental health researchers from the University of Michigan have recently calculated that approximately 90 percent of episodes of depression are due directly to stressful life events. It also appears that lower levels of sex hormones (estrogen and testosterone in women and testosterone in men) can exacerbate the depressive effects of cortisol during middle age. Researchers in Sweden have further shown that women with stress-related depression have increased levels of cortisol and IL-6 (a marker of inflammation from immune cells), suggesting that depression might also affect immune function.

It is interesting (and confusing) to note that a number of studies have shown cortisol levels to be *low* in people suffering from post-traumatic stress disorder (PTSD), while an equal number of studies have shown *high* cortisol levels in PTSD. Still other studies show no difference in cortisol levels between PTSD sufferers and "normal" individuals. Whether cortisol levels are high or low, it is clear that people with PTSD have many of the same day-to-day complaints as people suffering from "everyday" stress, including memory problems, sleep disturbances, daytime fatigue, and abdominal weight gain. Dutch researchers studying the similarities between PTSD and burnout have found many of the same levels of exhaustion, cynicism, feelings of reduced competence, and reduced cortisol levels—but they have also found that psychotherapeutic intervention (such as stress-management therapy) leads to a significant reduction in complaints and to an increase in cortisol levels back toward normal values (from suppressed levels). Neurobiology researchers in California have shown that cortisol is both good and bad for memory and overall brain function. At low levels, cortisol actually helps with memory formation and with retrieval of stored memories, but at *very* low levels (as in some cases of PTSD), or at high levels (as in cases of extreme or chronic stress), cortisol has been shown to interfere with the brain's ability to store new memories and recall old ones.

When it comes to extending what we know about cortisol's effects on the brain in terms of mood, anxiety, and depression to other brain abnormalities, it is tempting to speculate about the role of stress in Alzheimer's disease. It is important to note, however, that while there may be some superficial associations between high stress levels and Alzheimer's disease, we simply have no *direct* evidence that cortisol *causes* Alzheimer's disease, although chronic stress and elevated cortisol levels certainly appear able to make the situation much worse. It is true that most of us past the age of forty will begin to experience some degree of "normal" age-related memory loss (often called *age-related cognitive decline* or ARCD), but this is a far cry from the severe mental deterioration (senile dementia) usually seen with Alzheimer's disease. Although Alzheimer's disease may affect as many as 50 percent of people over age eighty-five to a certain degree, the condition involves a whole lot more than simple forgetfulness. Studies of the brain neurons from Alzheimer's patients show a clear pattern of death and destruction of cells in the parts of the brain involved in memory and higher thoughts.

It is also interesting, in light of our discussions of depression and anxiety, to note that Alzheimer's disease frequently begins with damage to the brain cells that produce a neurotransmitter called *acetylcholine*. The loss of acetylcholine causes symptoms ranging from the subtle, such as trouble remembering names or dates, to the more noticeable behavioral problems, such as depression and anxiety, and eventually to extreme disorientation and a loss of ability care for oneself. Drug treatment with Cognex or Aricept, which increase acetylcholine action, can produce a modest improvement in mild cases of Alzheimer's disease, but no existing drugs are able to restore normal function to the damaged regions of the brain.

So, stress and cortisol are erasing your memory, dashing your emotions, causing you anxiety, and killing your brain cells. Yikes! But you can do something about it. There are lots of steps you can take to make positive impacts on your stress response, on your cortisol levels, and on your feelings of depression and anxiety. That's what the next several chapters are about.

CORTISOL AND YOUR GUT

The image of stress-induced ulcers has been with us for decades. You've probably seen, on a TV sitcom or other such venue, the stereotypical portrayal of the stressed-out executive. Deadlines loom, stress builds, and the businessman gulps down antacids to quell the burning ulcer in his stomach. Far from being one of the many Hollywood overexaggerations, the phenomenon of stress-induced ulcers and other digestive problems has been documented in the medical literature for more than fifty years. From a physiological point of view, we know quite clearly that any stressful event will cause digestion to cease. Blood flow is diverted from the digestive organs to the heart and muscles, secretion of saliva and digestive enzymes is slowed, and intestinal contractions and absorption of nutrients stop. This rapid shutdown of the digestive process makes perfect sense, because from the standpoint of long-term survival it is more important to get away from the dangerous stressor (the lion) than to fully digest all your food. There will be plenty of time for digestion later; right now you need to save your skin. It is interesting to note, however, that even while stress hormones are signaling the body to shut down digestion, these same hormones, when kept elevated for more than a few minutes, are telling us to eat —and eat a lot!

Medical evidence shows quite clearly that ulcers of the stomach (gastric ulcers) and intestine (duodenal ulcers) are much more common in people who are anxious, depressed, or under chronic or repeated stress. In the face of these conditions, which are all also examples of chronic stressors, many of the digestive actions are curtailed, and the body also backs off from its production of other protective measures—such as the mucus that lines the stomach, and the bicarbonate that counteracts the highly acidic gastric juices. Sounds logical, right? And it is. Why should the body take a lot of protective measures against acid that will never be secreted (because you're under stress)? The problems start to occur when a person experiences the repeated cycles of high stress followed by low/normal stress that have become commonplace in our modern society. This sets up the digestive system for total confusion. Most of the time the body won't be able to secrete enough digestive enzymes to properly digest food (producing nausea, constipation, gas, and bloating). During the "lucky" times when a body *can* secrete enough digestive enzymes to properly break down food, the protective mechanisms are far from fully operational—which puts a person at risk for damage to her gastrointestinal tract (because the enzymes digest the gut's lining in addition to digesting the food). This scenario says a lot about why several bouts of intense stress are known to cause more ulcers than a longer continuous period of heightened stress.

To compound the problem, other factors, such as immune-system function and the body's control of inflammation and wound healing, come into play. It is well described in the medical literature that both repeated periods of acute stress and continuous periods of chronic stress are associated with suppressed immune-system activity. This has a direct bearing on ulcer development, because less immune-system activity means more growth and higher activity of a bacterium called *Helicobacter pylori*, which infects the stomach and causes ulcers in 80 percent of the people infected with it. Compounding the tissue damage caused by the accelerated growth of *H. pylori* is a suppression of the body's ability to heal that tissue damage because of an inhibition in prostaglandin synthesis. Prostaglandins are typically produced in response to tissue damage, where they help reduce inflammation and accelerate healing. During times of stress, however, the synthesis of prostaglandins is curtailed, which suggests that stress not only increases the rate at which ulcers may form, but also slows the rate at which they are repaired.

Aside from ulcers, the most common stress-related gut disease may be irritable bowel syndrome (IBS). Most of us will experience some degree of IBS during our lifetime. The name "IBS" is really a catchall for a variety of intestinal disorders, including colitis (inflammation of the lining of the large intestine, also known as the colon), in which abdominal pain is accompanied by diarrhea and/ or constipation, bloating, gas, and, occasionally, passing of mucus or blood. The majority of the gastrointestinal conditions falling under the IBS umbrella are either caused by or exacerbated by periods of heightened stress. Irish researchers have solidified the link between stress, inflammation, and gastrointestinal diseases such as IBS through a series of experiments involving 151 subjects that showed IBS to be clearly exacerbated by stressful psychological events, with cortisol and inflammatory cytokines such as IL-6 and IL-8 elevated in all forms of IBS (that is, IBS with diarrhea, IBS with constipation, and IBS with both).

So, again, we have bad news about stress and cortisol for an important bodily system. Stress leads to poor digestion, ulcerated stomachs, and inflamed intestines—not a pretty picture. These effects tend to result in poor dietary choices, suboptimal nutritional status, and a drop in energy levels and overall feelings of well-being. Getting stress and cortisol levels under control can help to reverse these problems.

CORTISOL, CONNECTIVE TISSUE, OSTEOPOROSIS, AND ARTHRITIS

Aging, as most of us know all too well, is associated with dramatic changes in some of the structural aspects of our bodies, such as bone and muscle strength, skin elasticity, and joint function. Profound changes in body composition also accompany advancing age,

so we progressively gain fat but lose muscle (sarcopenia), bone (os-
teopenia/osteoporosis), and joint cartilage (arthropenia/arthritis).
This means we are likely to get weaker (due to having less muscle),
feel tired (due to reduced aerobic endurance), and lose our ability
to get around efficiently. Many people simply accept these changes
as inevitable effects of the normal aging process—but they're not.

Luckily, researchers are learning more and more about the
precise causes of age-related losses in connective tissues (muscle,
bone, cartilage, skin, hair, and nails). While the cause of the aging
of these tissues remains quite complex, scientists are narrowing
down the list of potential mediating factors—and once again elevated cortisol levels are implicated as one of the primary markers
for accelerating these tissue losses (along with low levels of anabolic hormones, such as estrogen in women and testosterone and
DHEA in men).

Also fortunate is the fact that age-related loss of connective
tissue can be reversed, even in individuals nearing a hundred years
of age. Regular exercise programs incorporating strength training,
with or without aerobic exercise, have been shown to preserve or increase amounts of muscle, bone, and cartilage in older adults, while
also improving their ability to be independent. In addition, dietary
factors such as maintaining a protein intake of up to one gram of
protein per pound of body weight (see Chapter 7 for more detailed
protein recommendations) and a calcium intake of at least fifteen
hundred milligrams per day are well known to lead to positive benefits in terms of maintaining muscle and bone mass with age.

The relationship between elevated cortisol levels and an accelerated loss of cartilage, bone, and muscle has been demonstrated in
numerous situations, including cases of people with Cushing's syndrome (where elevated cortisol results in severe osteoporosis and
arthritis) and anorexia nervosa (where elevated cortisol leads to
bone and muscle loss). Studies such as these have also determined
that curing these diseases, and thereby removing the source of excess cortisol production, also restores cartilage, bone, and muscle
tissues. In experimental studies, cortisol has been shown to decrease

levels of connective-tissue growth factors and inhibit the activity of bone-building cells (osteoblasts), muscle-building cells (satellite cells), and cartilage-building cells (chondrocytes). So here we have a situation in which excess cortisol levels not only accelerate the breakdown of connective tissues, but also interfere with the biochemical process of building and repairing those same tissues.

The same scenario of increased loss and suppressed repair is seen in related connective tissues, such as skin, hair, and nails. The actions of cortisol to enhance the catabolism (breakdown) of many forms of connective tissues are well documented in the medical literature, and while these problems may not be of the same health magnitude as osteoporosis, nobody wants to have dry skin, thin hair, and cracked fingernails.

Most of us who have passed the age of forty have probably begun losing substantial amounts of muscle, bone, and cartilage, and our skin is a far cry from the soft, smooth stuff we were born with. We start to see these declines in connective-tissue quantity and quality starting in our mid-thirties and early forties, and by the time we're in our seventies, we're down about 20 percent from where we were in our twenties. These losses have all sorts of implications for how strong we are, how many calories we burn, how much energy we have, how we feel, and how we look. Elevated levels of cortisol as we age have been implicated in the acceleration of connective-tissue destruction, while declining levels of estrogen (in women), testosterone (in men), and IGF-1 and growth hormone (in both sexes) are known to be part of our hampered ability to rebuild damaged tissue.

The ability to rebuild damaged tissue plays a role in alleviating certain chronic pain conditions. Researchers at the University of Michigan have found that cortisol levels alone explained 38 percent of the variation in pain among patients with fibromyalgia, while scientists in Hong Kong have shown that optimism is able to reduce cortisol levels and perception of pain to a greater degree than pessimism and that negative thoughts can increase cortisol and subjective pain.

Greek researchers at the Athens Medical School have shown that high stress and cortisol levels not only increase inflammation throughout the body (via higher levels of cytokines), but also suppress thyroid-hormone metabolism. Suppressed thyroid function results in reduced levels of the active T3 form of thyroid hormone (which helps to maintain the body's metabolic rate) and increased levels of inactive rT3 (reducing the number of calories the body burns). And, as if a rise in inflammatory cytokines weren't bad enough for causing an increase in your risk for heart disease, researchers from the University of Alberta have also shown that cytokines stimulate cortisol activation by HSD, and thus may serve as the primary signal for inflammation-induced abdominal fat gain.

The good news in terms of connective-tissue maintenance is that a series of studies conducted at Tufts University and Penn State University have shown dramatic benefits in countering the frailty that is associated with extreme muscle, cartilage, and bone loss in the elderly. Results from these studies show that frail elderly participants are able to increase muscle and bone mass and *double* their muscle strength with resistance training performed two to three times a week. Participants in the exercise programs were able to get around more easily and with less joint pain than they could prior to the training. An interesting side benefit of the added muscle was an average 15 percent increase in daily caloric expenditure when compared to sedentary participants.

It's a bit harder to assess the effects of elevated cortisol levels on other connective tissues in humans, such as skin, hair, and nails. However, laboratory studies have shed some interesting light on the fact that excess cortisol bears a wide range of adverse effects on the underlying biochemistry of the skin and related tissues. For example, researchers in Finland have shown that while a low level of cortisol is able to stimulate the synthesis and slow the breakdown (by about 25 percent) of structural skin elements such as hyaluronan and proteoglycans, higher levels of cortisol have exactly the opposite effect, reducing synthesis and accelerating degradation of these compounds by more than 40 percent. Both hyaluronan and proteoglycans are responsible for hydrating the skin by attracting and holding adequate amounts of moisture, so reduced levels of these compounds in the skin mean that the skin dries out. Similar effects have been noted for related skin proteins, such as elastin (needed for skin elasticity) and collagen (needed for skin strength), and these observations have led many researchers to hypothesize that elevated cortisol levels may be responsible for accelerated skin "aging" and the overall skin atrophy (wrinkling) observed during drug treatment with synthetic cortisol.

CORTISOL AND AGING

Although you can't do anything about your age, it is probably important to discuss the differences in stress response between younger and older people. In very general terms, it appears to be true that as we age, we become less able to deal effectively with stress. This means that for the same "load" of stress, whether from exercise, illness, emotions, or whatever, a younger person will tend to "deal better" with the stressor compared to an older person. The primary difference does not seem to be much of a difference in the initial response to the stressor; old folks tend to secrete just as many stress hormones as their younger counterparts (though older folks also tend to have higher cortisol levels even under normal, nonstressed conditions). Instead, younger subjects tend to recover faster from stress, so they're able to get their cortisol levels back to within normal ranges in a much shorter period of time compared to older subjects. Being able to quickly turn off the stress response following the removal of a given stressor also appears to be associated with a slower growth of cancer cells (tumors), so the youngsters appear to have an edge when it comes to fending off cancer (at least in lab rats).

To better understand the relationship between cortisol and aging, let's consider the situation of the salmon. You probably know the basics of the story: The salmon swims upstream for thousands of miles, spawns, and quickly dies. (Some life!) If you were to catch a salmon right after spawning, you'd see a few interesting things, such as a poor immune system, lots of infections, unhealed wounds, stomach ulcers, etc. Sounds like an overactive stress response—and that's exactly what it is. Marine biologists have studied the physiology of spawning salmons to find that, lo and behold, they have outrageously high cortisol levels. Take it one step further and remove the adrenal glands from these salmon, and guess what happens? Having no adrenal glands means that the salmon experience no cortisol secretion and no rapid onset of death; they live on perfectly well for another year or so (which is quite a long time for a fish). The primary reason why cortisol levels go completely crazy in salmon is that they rapidly develop an inability to regulate their cortisol secretion. For some reason, their bodies fail to recognize the fact that they have plenty of cortisol in their system, so the adrenals just keep churning out more and more—and every organ system quickly deteriorates. A similar age-related breakdown in the regulation of cortisol secretion occurs in other animals, including mice, rats, dogs, monkeys, baboons, and humans (though none quite as dramatically as in the salmon).

One of the most exciting findings in the last few years of stress research has been that made by scientists at the University of California at San Francisco. Researchers in the Department of Psychiatry there have shown a distinct link between psychological stress and accelerated rates of aging in humans. For years, we've known that stress causes rodents, worms, and baboons to age faster, but this is the first direct evidence we have to indicate faster aging in stressed people—and, as you might expect, increased rates of high cholesterol, high blood pressure, high blood sugar, and greater abdominal obesity.

In a study of teachers in Finland, older teachers (average age fifty-four) were found to have much higher cortisol exposure and elevated blood pressure compared to younger teachers (average age thirty-one). The difference in cortisol levels was found to be due to the older teachers' inability to "recover" from high levels of job stress. Both younger and older groups had high cortisol levels at work, but only the younger teachers showed a reduced cortisol level after work. Stanford University psychiatrists have shown that caregivers of chronically ill patients (whether professional or family caregivers) have significantly higher levels of cortisol, which may be related to development of mental dysfunction in later life.

Italian researchers have shown that the older we get, the more cortisol we have, and the worse memory. These researchers have indicated that the cortisol/age/memory relationship is largely due to cortisol's tendency to shrink an area of the brain called the *hippocampus,* which has a high level of cortisol receptors and is involved in memory. Not only did levels of cortisol in the research subjects grow higher with age, but levels of testosterone fell, leading to a "double-whammy" detrimental effect on brain function with age. British researchers from the Birmingham University Medical School have also shown that as cortisol levels go up and testosterone levels fall with age and stress, immune function also falls, leading to an increase in infection rates in stressed elderly people.

So does this mean we're all destined to succumb to cortisol-related organ failure as we age? Certainly not. Making some of the right choices in terms of exercise regimen, dietary intake, sleep patterns, and the judicious use of nutritional supplements can go a long way toward retarding some of what we now view as "age-related" changes in how our bodies work and how we look and feel.

SUMMARY

Whew! If the preceding information doesn't stress you out (even a little bit), then you haven't been reading very closely. At first glance, many of us might view the close relationship between stress, cortisol, and the long list of chronic diseases as a hopeless disaster just waiting to happen—and for a great many people, it is. The good news, however, is that armed with the right information and the proper motivation, one can do a great deal to counteract these potential problems. The general idea is to control the stress response in such a way that cortisol levels are maintained within their optimal range—not too high and not too low—with long-term health and wellness as the outcome. The rest of the book shows you how.

CHAPTER 7

Counteracting the Effects of Chronic Stress

sk almost anybody about their stress level and you're bound to hear that it's high (unless you tend to surround yourself with Type B, laid-back folks, like Californian surfers). Enduring a high level of stress is almost a badge of honor these days; if you don't claim to be under extreme stress, then you might feel that others will view you as somewhat of a slacker.

Okay, so let's accept the fact that most of us have plenty of stress to deal with. Is this necessarily a bad thing? No, because some people can handle a great deal of stress without succumbing to any of its detrimental health effects—at least for a period of time. Some people even claim to thrive on stress, when we know that what they really thrive on is the jolt of adrenaline and endorphins stressful situations cause their bodies to produce. Unfortunately, while adrenaline and endorphins will certainly pump us up with energy and good feelings (at least for a few minutes), the resulting cortisol secretion can get us into health trouble over the long term.

But how do you know if all this applies to you? How do you know where you stand on the stress spectrum? How do you know if you're at risk for all the nasty health problems outlined in the preceding chapters? Simple. Refer back to the results of your Type C

Self-Test, located in the Introduction. (If you haven't yet taken the test, totaled your results, and discovered your Type C index, now is a good time to take a few minutes and do so.) Chances are, you are a Stressed Jess. That means everything in this book—from the warnings about the effects of excessive stress and increased cortisol levels, to the advice about how you can counteract those effects—applies to you.

But even if you're not always a Stressed Jess, there are almost certainly times when a Strained Jane or a Relaxed Jack could use a helping hand with stress management. Whether you're a hard-charging Type A go-getter or a more relaxed, roll-with-the-punches Type B, we are all periodically at risk for slipping into the Type C lifestyle (which is characterized by elevated cortisol levels). For the Janes and Jacks out there, this book can be used as an a la carte resource: Try a bit of this and a little of that to see which cortisol-control strategies work most effectively for your particular situation.

ADRENAL STRESS TESTING KITS

Should you run out and purchase one of those at-home kits that measure cortisol levels in saliva or urine? Probably not. Although quite a cottage industry has sprung up to sell you home hormone-testing kits, the validity and utility of such kits are limited—and the same goes for the more sophisticated hormone analysis that can be ordered by your doctor. Why? The main reason these tests are unnecessary for most people is because levels of cortisol, DHEA, testosterone, and related hormones fluctuate normally throughout the day and can change at a moment's notice. This means that the very act of taking the test is likely to change the results, making them virtually useless unless administered in just the right way, which is very difficult even under controlled laboratory conditions.

We perform measurements of both cortisol and testosterone in our nutrition clinic as part of our SENSE Lifestyle Program, but we do this in a research setting to quantify the magnitude of hormone control across groups of participants—not to classify them as having "high" or "low" levels of a particular hormone. In most cases, you'll already know whether you're experiencing heightened stress. By answering the questions in the Type C Self-Test (which we also use in our studies of the SENSE program), you can get a very good idea of how much stress you're exposed to, how you tend to deal with that stress, and what level of risk that stress may pose for your long-term health. (You'll also save yourself the $100 to $400 that is typically charged for the mail-order adrenal stress tests.)

CONTROLLING THE STRESS RESPONSE: THE SENSE LIFESTYLE PROGRAM

Some of the best news contained in this book is the fact that there are almost as many different ways to *deal* with stress as there are things that *cause* stress. We all know the basics for coping with stress (Grandma has been telling us for years), but we often forget just how effective some of those simple remedies really can be. Perhaps the most effective antistress activities are also the easiest to accomplish. Practices such as eating a balanced diet, getting adequate rest, and performing some regular exercise can do wonders for helping the body adapt and respond to stressful events. Unfortunately, stress often causes us to do just the opposite: We eat junk food, we can't seem to relax, and we have no time for exercise, each of which only serves to compound the problem and exacerbate the detrimental effects of stress on our bodies. Controlling your individual stress response with various relaxation techniques can help to modulate cortisol secretion and normalize metabolism, but for many people such techniques simply are unrealistic in the face of their hectic lifestyles. So what to do?

We already know from the preceding chapters that controlling cortisol levels will yield all sorts of wonderful health benefits. Returning cortisol to an optimal range will return caloric expenditure back to normal, reduce body fat, preserve muscle mass, decrease appetite, and increase energy levels—and these are just some of the effects you'll be able to *feel*. Other benefits of controlling cortisol levels—such as reducing cholesterol and blood sugar, maintaining brain power, reducing bone loss, and strengthening immune function—will occur more "silently," meaning you're still reaping the benefits but you won't necessarily notice them in the same way as you will an increased energy level or a slimmer waistline.

To reduce the incidence of certain diseases, the use of behavioral interventions that decrease stress can be just as beneficial for long-term health as quitting smoking, losing weight, reducing cholesterol levels, eating well, or exercising. In other words, if it's possible to avoid stressful situations, then that is the obvious first course of action. Unfortunately, avoiding stress is not always possible or realistic for most of us. Therefore, either you need to learn how to deal with stress as effectively as possible—often referred to as *stress management*—or you need to find a way to reduce the effects of stress on your body.

The hard part, of course, is deciding on the best approach to controlling cortisol levels for *you*. For some people, a stress-management approach, such as practicing relaxation techniques, is the most appropriate method for controlling cortisol, while others may prefer to exercise their cortisol levels into normal ranges, and still others may turn to dietary supplements as a convenient way to get cortisol levels under control.

The sections that follow summarize a program of general recommendations for controlling cortisol levels. This approach is called the SENSE program. SENSE stands for **S**tress management, **E**xercise, **N**utrition, **S**upplements, and **E**valuation—the five key areas that can be readily acted upon by anyone to control cortisol levels. (This chapter summarizes the first four parts of the program, S, E, N, and S. Evaluation, the second "E" in SENSE, is covered in Chapter 9.) As you read

The SENSE Program
S = Stress management
E = Exercise
N = Nutrition
S = Supplements
E = Evaluation

through the rest of this chapter and the chapters to come, keep in mind that the SENSE Lifestyle Program is a research-proven approach to controlling your body's stress response to help you lose weight and feel a whole lot better. SENSE has been conducted and studied for more than five years and has been presented at some of the top nutrition-science conferences in the world, including the American College of Nutrition, Experimental Biology, the American College of Sports Medicine, the International Society for Sports Nutrition, and the North American Society for the Study of Obesity. Across these presentations, the average results for participants just like you have shown significant drops in body-fat levels, maintenance of hormone profiles, control of cholesterol, and dramatic improvements in mood and energy levels—and we do all of this with a phenomenally high completion rate (90 percent of our participants complete the SENSE program, compared to the typical 50 percent completion rate for many commercial and diet-book programs). For more detailed coverage of the topics of diet, exercise, relaxation, and other stress-management techniques, numerous excellent books are available; see the Resources section in the back of this book for some recommendations. See also Chapter 9, devoted entirely to the SENSE program.

STRESS MANAGEMENT AND AVOIDANCE (OR WHERE DID OUR VACATIONS GO?)

A recent study by the Families and Work Institute gave us some very bad news—one in three American workers felt chronically overworked. The culprit? Technology—mostly those items like cell phones, Blackberries, and e-mail that enable us to be working anywhere and everywhere—and, unfortunately, all the time. It's really too bad that "being busy" has become such a status symbol (damn that Puritan work ethic), because it is clear from the scientific research that being too busy and always being "on" is detrimental to long-term physical and mental health. Don't get me wrong—hard work is both important and valuable, but working too hard for too long leads to burnout, reduced creativity, and inefficiency.

Ideas and theories abound concerning the management of stress and the modulation of the stress response. Many of these ideas revolve around some aspect of regaining "control" over the stress response, typically by attempting to control the degree of stress or make the stressor occur with predictability. Why should this make any difference—after all, a stressor is a stressor, right? Maybe not. For example, *any* lion charging at you from the bushes is going to be stressful, but knowing *where* and *when* that lion will charge may make the stress a bit more manageable.

We know from studies of both animals and humans that at least three factors can make a huge difference in how the body responds to a given stressor: whether there is any *outlet* for the stress, whether the stressor is *predictable,* and whether the human or animal thinks they have any *control* over the stressor. These three factors—outlet, predictability, and control—emerge as modulating factors again and again in research studies of stress. For example, put a rat in a cage and subject it to a series of low-voltage electric shocks (sounds pretty stressful), and the rat gets elevated cortisol levels and develops ulcers (you would too). Take another rat, give it the same series of shocks, but also give it an outlet for its stress—such as something to chew on, something to eat, or a wheel to run on—and its cortisol levels do not go up (as much) and it does not get ulcers. The same is true for humans under stress: Go for a run, scream at the wall, or do something else that serves as an outlet for controlling cortisol levels—and cortisol levels are reduced (somewhat) and many of the detrimental effects of stress are counteracted (or at least modulated).

Let's turn now to the second of the three stress modulators, predictability. Let's say that somebody woke you up in the middle of the night, put you on a plane, and then made you jump out of it at ten thousand feet. Pretty stressful, huh? This experience would certainly be accompanied by elevated heart rate and blood pressure, changes in blood levels of glucose and fatty acids, and, of course, a huge increase in blood cortisol levels. What do you think would happen if you were forced to do this every other night or so for the next few months? Far from being a stressed-out bundle of nerves, you would actually get accustomed to it—and your stress response would become less pronounced. This scenario has actually been studied in army rangers training at jump school to become paratroopers. At the start of training, the soldiers underwent enormous increases in cortisol levels during each jump, but by the end of the course, their stress responses were virtually nonexistent. By making the stressor more predictable, the stress response of each soldier was controlled to a much greater degree (though skydiving will probably never become a completely stress-free activity).

Finally, the concept of control is central to understanding why some people respond to a stressor with gigantic elevations in cortisol, while others respond to the same stressor with a much lower cortisol response. This concept has been demonstrated in rats that have been trained to press a lever to avoid getting shocked. Every time the rat gets shocked, it presses the lever, and the next shock is delayed for several minutes. If that lever is then made nonoperational, so it has no effect on the timing of the next shock, the rats still have a lower occurrence of stress-related diseases (such as ulcers and infections) because they *think* they still have control over the shocks. An interesting comparison can be made to people working under high-stress conditions, such as during a period of corporate layoffs. For many workers, this situation is one of high instability and low control (thus high stress), while for others, perhaps those in a department that will be unaffected by job cuts, there is much less stress (and fewer health problems).

This third stress modulator, one's feeling of being in control, does *not* mean that you need to try to gain a high degree of control over every aspect of your life—because trying to do so can actually *increase* your cortisol levels. Instead, for most of us, it means doing your best, as the saying goes, to control those things you can control and to accept those things you cannot change (or have no control over).

Swiss researchers at the University of Zurich's Institute of Psychology have shown that stress-management techniques can reduce stress, anxiety, and cortisol exposure in "real-life" stressful situations. According to the researchers, the importance of daily stress management cannot be overemphasized because of the findings that long-term chronic stress exposure (and high cortisol) can eventually lead to an inability to mount a normal stress response (and, thus, to a suppressed cortisol level). Canadian psychology researchers at the Alberta Cancer Board have shown that "mindfulness-based stress reduction" (yoga, meditation, and relaxation exercises) results in a rapid and dramatic improvement in overall quality of life, symptoms of stress, and sleep quality in women with breast cancer and men with prostate cancer. German researchers have shown that people in chronic-stress states can benefit from *simplified* stress-management approaches, such as weekly yoga classes, which result in improvements in cortisol levels and psychological measures of stress, well-being, vigor, fatigue, and depression.

At this point in the book, it should go without saying that managing your stress response is a good thing—but the fact remains that most of us will not bother to follow that advice. However, incorporating some stress management into your life doesn't necessarily mean locking yourself in a dark room in order to get in touch with your inner self. Rather, it first involves understanding that you have stress in your life (easy) and accepting that stress will do "bad things" to your body and health (also easy) unless you do something about it (easier than you think). Luckily, there are a great many techniques, several of them research-based, that you can use to help manage your body's stress response—and many of them don't even involve drastic lifestyle changes. For example, consider the following:

Change your e-mail program so it checks for new messages only once per hour. Most e-mail programs are set to check for new messages every five minutes. This means you're interrupted by the new-message beep ninety-six times in an eight-hour day! How do you expect to get any "real" work done? Also, consider (as I do) shutting *off* your e-mail program until the second half of your day, which will enable you to get your "important" work accomplished in the morning when you're mentally fresh.

Whenever possible, leave the cell phone behind. Even if you tell yourself that you won't answer it, there is a part of your mind that is waiting for the ring. You need to let that part of your brain relax and forget about the phone at least every now and then.

Read trash. Get a book or magazine that has no redeeming social value—and enjoy it. If this is too decadent for your tastes, then alternate a "good" book that might teach you something with a "junk" book that you can simply lose yourself in. Why? Because it allows your mind to "escape" and recharge, so it comes back even stronger, more creative, and more resilient to stress. On a recent cross-country flight I sat next to a woman who was reading a genetic research journal. (I was reading a bicycling magazine.) As a fellow scientist, I commented on her reading material, and she laughed because underneath her research journal she had one of those celebrity-gossip tabloids that you see at the grocery checkout stand. She explained that she couldn't wait to "get through" her genetics journal so she could "catch up" on the latest "dirt"—it was hilarious. It turns out that we were both headed to the same obesity research conference in Boston, and we both appreciated the importance of "getting away" for a few minutes in our magazines.

Take daily mini-vacations. I do a lot of sitting in front of a computer, but I also get up every hour or two for a quick stretch or a walk around the office. You'll be amazed at how a quick flex of your muscles and a surge in your circulation can help to clear the cobwebs from your mind. One of the best ways to de-stress during your workday is to revive the lost art of lunch. Take it! Too may people skip lunch (bad metabolically and mentally) or gobble it down at their desks (which is even worse). Instead, take the hour to enjoy a healthy meal and relax your mind. Even better, use that hour to visit with friends or coworkers—you'll have a more productive second half of the day and likely accomplish even more high-quality work with improved creativity and efficiency than if you had worked through lunch.

Take a full day off each week. No work. No thoughts about work or worries about work. Take this day to rest and reflect and re-charge (whether or not a "Sabbath" day has any religious connota-tions for you). Read a book. Take a walk. Luxuriate in the act of doing nothing. I guarantee that if you give yourself over to a solid month of "do-nothing Sundays," you will feel more physically and mentally refreshed than you could possible imagine. Doing nothing will give you back a lot.

Recreate to re-create. Giving yourself permission to relax does not mean that you're a slacker; it means that you're a step ahead of the nose-to-the-grindstone automatons who are on a fast road to burnout. As a long-time nutrition consultant to some of the world's top athletes, I can tell you without question that knowing when to go hard and when to ease off is what separates Olympic champi-ons from also-rans. While your own life might be "too busy" most of the time, it is those moments of relaxation and decompression that allow you to keep jumping back in with renewed energy and creativity.

Get a massage. Australian researchers have shown that something as simple as a fifteen-minute weekly back massage reduced cortisol levels, blood pressure, and overall measures of anxiety in a group of high-stress nurses. Another study of massage conducted at the University of Miami School of Medicine showed a remarkable 31 percent reduction in cortisol levels following massage therapy, as well as a 28 percent increase in the feel-good neurotransmitter se-rotonin.

Take a bath. Japanese scientists in Osaka have shown a significant reduction in cortisol levels in high-stress men following a relaxing hot bath. The men with the highest stress levels had the most dra-matic reductions in cortisol levels.

Imagine creative solutions. Japanese researchers in Kyoto have shown that guided-imagery exercises (relaxing by imagining solu-tions to stress) can reduce cortisol levels after the very first session.

In a series of studies, subjects practiced replacing unpleasant mental images of stressful events with comfortable thoughts, resulting in a displacement of stress, a shift toward a balanced emotional state, and a significant drop in cortisol exposure. Psychology researchers at UCLA have also shown that stressed patients who perform a "value affirmation task" (mentally reciting their personal values) in reaction to stressful events are able to reduce their cortisol responses to stress. Remember *The Little Engine That Could?* Well, little children show the same resilience to stress when they apply the "I think I can" approach to school stressors. In a study by Swedish researchers, school kids had lower cortisol levels when they approached stressful situations with mental imagery that affirmed, "I can solve this task."

Take a long weekend. Even short periods of getting away can result in a significant drop in cortisol levels. In one study, a three-day, two-night weekend led to a decrease in cortisol levels and overall stress markers as well as a boost in immune-system function.

Take a yoga class. Swedish psychologists have recently shown that ten sessions of yoga over four weeks results in significant benefits in psychology and physiology in both men and women. Participants in the yoga sessions had improvements in cortisol, stress, anger, exhaustion, and blood pressure levels.

Pray. Research on religion at Arizona State University has shown that people who are more spiritual and pray more often have lower cortisol levels and lower blood pressure.

Get a pet. Scientists at Virginia Commonwealth University want you to get a dog. Based on their findings, high-stress health-care professionals were able to significantly lower their cortisol levels after as little as five minutes of "dog therapy." Though there were no measures of cortisol levels in the pooches, we can imagine that they also benefited from playing with the health-care workers.

Crank up the tunes. French scientists showed that relaxing music was able to significantly reduce cortisol levels following a stressful event (as compared to silence).

Get some sleep. Getting enough sleep is far and away the most effective stress-management technique that we have available to us. Did you know that as little as a night or two of good, sound, restful sleep may do more for controlling your cortisol levels and reducing your long-term risk for many chronic diseases than a whole lifetime of stress-management classes? The importance of adequate sleep for controlling your stress response, helping you lose weight, boosting your energy levels, and improving your mood cannot be overemphasized. Here's why.

When you were just a few months old, a mere babe, your brain had you programmed to sleep about eighteen hours a day—not a very stressful existence. Upon reaching adulthood—at say approximately twenty years of age—your nightly allotment of sleep had been slashed to less than seven hours (six hours and fifty-four minutes, according to the National Sleep Foundation). That's approximately two hours less than the eight to nine hours recommended by sleep experts for optimal physical and mental health. Progressive changes in your brain's internal clock (the suprachiasmatic nucleus), combined with alterations in your patterns of hormone secretion, have you going to bed later and waking up earlier with each successive decade, resulting in nearly thirty minutes less sleep per night with every ten years you age. By the time we reach our thirties and forties, we're getting 80 percent less time in the most restful "slow-wave" period of sleep (as compared to our teenage years), and by the time we hit our fifties and sixties, we get almost no uninterrupted deep sleep. (We still get *some* deep sleep, but it tends to come in short fragments that do little in terms of recovery and repair for mind and body.)

What does this lack of sleep mean for your cortisol levels? It means that the average fifty-year-old has nighttime cortisol levels more than twelve times higher than the average thirty-year-old—yikes! Perhaps the worst piece of news is that not only will an inadequate quality or quantity of sleep result in elevated cortisol levels, but high cortisol will also limit both your ability to fall asleep and the amount of time that your mind spends in the most restful stages of deep sleep. This sets you up for a vicious cycle of poor sleep, elevated cortisol, and subtle changes in metabolism that leads you down the path toward chronic diseases.

A study from Yale University of 1,709 men found that those who regularly got less than six hours of shut-eye doubled their risk of weight gain and diabetes because of excess cortisol exposure and its interference with insulin metabolism and blood-sugar control. A similar study at Columbia University showed that sleeping less than five hours nightly was associated with twice the risk of high blood pressure.

Researchers from the University of Virginia have found that jet lag—and the elevated stress and cortisol that come from sleep deprivation and altered body-clock cycles—is not just bad for health, but can lead to higher death rates as well (at least in older mice). The increased death rates are thought to be due to a suppression of immune-system function caused by elevated cortisol levels (but the simple fact that sleep-deprived mice die sooner probably comes as no surprise to exhausted, globe-trotting business executives or stretched-to-the-limit soccer moms).

Researchers at Brown University Medical School have recently shown that sleep *quality* (how *restful* your sleep is), but not necessarily sleep *quantity* (how many hours of sleep you get), is closely related to cortisol exposure. As you might imagine, subjects with lower levels of sleep quality (including children and teenagers) also had the highest cortisol exposure and a higher degree of overall stress. In a related series of experiments by researchers at the National Institute for Psychosocial Medicine, in Stockholm, Sweden, total sleep time was significantly decreased (and sleepiness and cortisol increased) in workers during their most stressful workweeks (no surprise there). The stress at work in these subjects also led to daytime sleepiness—but even though the workers were tired, they were still too stressed to sleep at night.

Researchers at Stanford University's Sleep Disorders Clinic have recently shown that cortisol can affect "slow-wave" sleep, interrupting the deeper (most restful) stages of sleep and setting the stage for increased risk of developing diabetes, high blood pressure, depression, insomnia, and obesity later in life. A related sleep study from UCLA suggests that cortisol overexposure reduces deep-sleep delta waves and in doing so further increases cortisol levels and sets the stage for higher risk of PTSD in susceptible individuals.

Swedish sleep researchers in Stockholm have recently shown that the number of "micro-arousals" (quick wakeups that you might not even be aware of) from sleep is closely related to cortisol levels—with more arousals increasing cortisol exposure. The researchers found that the number of micro-arousals was related to the degree of work-related stress—with more work stress related to a higher number of nightly micro-arousals. As is the case with other forms of sleep loss and sleep fragmentation, micro-arousals were associated with metabolic indicators suggestive of a higher risk for obesity and diabetes. In a related series of sleep experiments by German scientists, helicopter pilots with reduced sleep levels (cutting sleep time from 7.8 hours to 6 hours or less nightly) were found to have elevations in cortisol exposure amounting to up to 80 percent—with elevated levels persisting even after two nights of full-duration sleep.

Some of the most disturbing evidence citing sleep deprivation as a major source of stress comes from University of Chicago sleep researchers. In a study presented at the American Diabetes Association Annual Scientific Conference, the Chicago group found that inadequate sleep leads to increased cortisol levels, insulin resistance and higher blood-sugar levels, elevated appetite, and weight gain. The scariest part of the study was that the "normal" sleepers averaged 7.5 to 8.5 hours of sleep per night, while the sleep-deprived "short" sleepers were only missing out on an hour or two of nightly shut-eye (averaging about 6.5 hours of sleep per night). Simply losing a few hours of sleep resulted in a 50 percent increase in cortisol exposure and a 40 percent reduction in insulin function.

How many of us feel *lucky* to get seven hours of sleep? I know I do—yet I know this is not enough sleep to keep my cortisol exposure as low as I want it to be. I also know that some of the best ways to ensure a restful night of sleep are to avoid caffeine after noon (yet I sit here writing this at 3:00 P.M. with a cup of java next to the laptop), leave work at the office (yet I'm writing this from my home office), and skip the late-night TV (yet my Tivo lets me watch primetime shows after I put the kids to bed)—so that's three strikes for me. How many strikes do you have against your ability to get enough restful shut-eye? (See Chapter 9 for some specific pointers that will help you get more sleep.)

I tell you all of this because it is important for you to understand that following the SENSE program is not an "all or nothing" proposition. Sometimes you'll have lots of stress, and sometimes you'll have less. Some of the time you might get adequate sleep; much of the time you won't. On certain days you'll be able to exercise hard and eat right—and on other days you'll hit the drive-through and feel like you live at the office. The point here is not to strive to be perfect in your approach to making SENSE out of your stressful life, but rather to do as much as you can whenever you can without the program becoming yet another source of stress in your life.

The next three sections of this chapter concern exercise, nutrition, and supplements—and it is these aspects that represent the heart of the program. Concentrate on these components to generate the most dramatic effects on your weight, mood, and energy levels.

EXERCISE

Being active can help reduce some of the detrimental effects of chronic cortisol exposure. Exercise leads to the production of dopamine and serotonin, both of which are "feel-good" antianxiety and antidepression chemicals that are produced in the brain and are responsible for the well-known effect of "runner's high" that can help control the stress response. Researchers at Duke University have shown that exercise (thirty minutes per day, three to four days a week, for four months) can be as effective as prescription antidepressants in relieving symptoms of anxiety and depression.

Researchers at the University of Colorado have conducted several studies that show how exercise can reduce many of the detrimental effects of chronic stress. Regular participation in *moderate* exercise can reduce body fat, build muscle and bone, improve mental and emotional function, stimulate the immune response, and reduce appetite. The Colorado researchers have also shown that *extremes* of exercise, such as that undertaken by overtrained endurance athletes, can reverse these benefits by elevating cortisol levels, increasing body fat, interfering with mental and emotional functioning, suppressing immune function, and increasing the risk of injury. Scientists at the National Institutes of Health have noted that regular exercise can help patients with extremely elevated cortisol levels (those with a condition known as Cushing's syndrome) prevent many of the metabolic derangements and much of the tissue destruction normally seen during the course of the disease. Stress researchers in Arizona have shown that being more physically fit is protective against stress and against the age-related rise in cortisol levels. The research findings show that older unfit women had significantly greater cortisol exposure in response to stress compared to young unfit women and older fit women. As expected, higher fitness reduced cortisol levels in both younger and older women and may be one reason why regular exercise helps to protect against many stress-related diseases.

It is important to understand that the exercise component of SENSE is less about burning calories (although that is a nice side benefit) and is intended more as a "metabolic hedge" against cortisol's tendency to reduce the body's metabolic rate. Previous chapters have discussed the roles of cortisol and testosterone in maintaining muscle mass and metabolic rate, but there are some other simple strategies for helping to keep your middle-aged metabolism from covering your midsection in fat—and regular exercise is one way to do that. Remember that metabolic rate starts slowing after about age twenty, so by the age of forty your ability to burn calories has dropped by about 10 percent. To prevent this metabolic drop, three of the most important (and simplest) things you can do include the following:

Never skip breakfast. Doing so can cause your metabolic rate to drop by 5 percent (further reducing your ability to burn calories) until you eat something. (More about nutrition in the next section.)

Lift weights one to two times weekly. Adding a single pound of new muscle to your frame means your body will burn an extra fifty calories every day, which is equivalent to burning five pounds of pure fat every year. Add five pounds of new muscle and you're looking at an automatic twenty-five-pound fat loss by this time next year.

Drink more water. Drinking just two extra glasses of H_2O per day can boost your metabolism by 30 percent. Most of us are slightly dehydrated anyway, which suppresses our metabolic rate, so those extra glasses are really just bringing our metabolic machinery back to optimal function—and accelerating fat loss in the process.

> *Josh,* a real estate agent, husband, and father of four, was a perfect candidate for developing many of the adverse health conditions associated with stress and elevated cortisol levels. Despite knowing that exercise would be a great outlet for his stress, Josh felt that his irregular work schedule (long hours, nights, and weekends) meant that he had no time for a regular exercise program. However, by treating his daily exercise as a "client" and actually scheduling time for it into his agenda, he was finally able to begin adhering to a regular program of jogging and lifting weights three times per week. Through exercise, Josh was able to harness his body's fight-or-flight hormonal system to help reduce stress and balance cortisol levels. The results for Josh have been most noticeable in terms of his energy levels and degree of creativity—both of which have impacted favorably on his real estate practice and his family life.

Good for Josh for managing to wedge a regular exercise regimen into his weekly schedule. But what about you? You may have joined gyms, tried jogging, and spent big bucks on fancy treadmills and stationary cycles that now serve mostly as coat racks—yet nothing seems to stick. (Hints for alternative ways to work some physical activity into your normal daily routine are included in Chapter

9. Additionally, check out the Resources section for books on the topic of exercise.)

NUTRITION

Eating right is also an important part of counteracting the effects of cortisol (big surprise). Proper diet can help modulate inflammatory responses in the body while also promoting tissue repair. When it comes to what a "proper" diet is, however, things can get a bit complicated—and it is unfortunate that so many people get truly stressed out about their diets, because they don't have to (and when they do, it causes problems). For example, Canadian nutrition researchers have shown in a number of studies that "cognitive dietary restraint" (CDR, or "a perceived ongoing effort to limit dietary intake to manage body weight"—what you know simply as "dieting") is a potent trigger for increasing cortisol and reducing bone mass in both young and older women. In studies of younger (premenopausal) women, the impact of stress and cortisol on bone loss was thought to be partly due to cortisol's disruption of menstrual cycles, but newer research from Texas Tech University shows that cortisol overexposure has a direct and rapid detrimental effect on bone (increasing bone breakdown) that is separate from effects on the menstrual cycle. In a group of older (postmenopausal) women, having higher levels of CDR resulted in cortisol levels that were almost 20 percent higher than in women with lower levels of CDR. Many excellent books have been written on the topic of optimizing diet (see the Resources section). Instead of rehashing these nutritional recommendations, the following general suggestions are presented to help you craft your own cortisol-controlling diet plan. In addition, the very simple and easy-to-follow "Helping Hand" approach to eating that we use in SENSE is outlined for you in Chapter 9.

What to Avoid?

One of the most positive antistress decisions you can make in terms of your diet is to cut down your use of alcohol, caffeine, and dietary supplements containing stimulants (such as ephedra). Does this mean you have to swear off any enjoyment of cola, coffee, tea, wine, chocolate, or beer? Certainly not, but it is important to understand that too much caffeine or related stimulants can send the already-stimulated nervous system from a state of heightened alertness into a state of nervousness and anxiety. In other people, alcohol can induce the same series of effects. Despite the fact that many people reach for a drink to calm their nerves (which it can do quite nicely), alcohol also acts as a diuretic to make the body lose water. This diuretic action often leaves a person in a dehydrated state, which the body perceives as a stressor, resulting in—you guessed it—elevated cortisol levels. Furthermore, alcohol can increase the occurrence of nighttime awakenings, an effect that is likely to counteract the otherwise restorative effects of sleep.

Dietary supplements targeted to weight loss and weight maintenance represent the largest category in the entire supplement industry. The key problem, however, is that many of the most popular dietary supplements on the market can actually increase cortisol levels in the body and make long-term weight control more difficult—primarily because they deliver an excessive dose of stimulants. Even though many of these supplements can be quite effective in suppressing appetite and increasing energy expenditure over a few short weeks (plenty of studies show this to be true), when used at high doses they also cause stress at the tissue and cellular levels. The body perceives this stimulant-mediated stress in the very same way that it perceives other forms of stress, and it responds by increasing the body's secretion of cortisol, which effectively sabotages any weight-loss successes experienced in the first few weeks of use. Taking supplements of this type can certainly help you lose weight, but when taken to excess they actually hurt your chances of long-term weight maintenance because of this effect of increasing cortisol levels.

Among the most important supplements to avoid at high doses are the herbal stimulants such as ma huang (ephedra), *Sida cordifolia* (ephedra), guarana (caffeine), *Citrus aurantium* (synephrine), coleus (forskolin), and yohimbe (yohimbine)—all of which increase the output of adrenaline and cortisol from the adrenal glands (and all of which are covered in more detail in the next chapter).

What to Eat?

We have the "what to avoid" part out of the way; now for the more interesting part about what to eat. When it comes to designing an antistress diet, the most important consideration is to maintain a balanced intake of the major macronutrients (protein, carbohydrates, and fats) along with the micronutrients (vitamins, minerals, and phytonutrients; see Chapter 8 for a detailed discussion of the role played by vitamins and minerals in combating the effects of stress and cortisol).

By selecting your blend of *macronutrients* from the "right" kinds of foods—brightly colored fruits and veggies teamed with whole grains and lean cuts of meat, poultry, and fish—the vast majority of your *micronutrient* needs will automatically be satisfied. For example, a balanced breakfast of a scrambled egg, a piece of whole-grain toast, and a glass of orange juice provides a powerful dose of antistress nutrients. It contains protein (in the egg), carbohydrates (in the toast and juice), B vitamins (in the toast), antioxidants (in the juice), and phytonutrients (carotenoid lutein in the egg, citrus bioflavonoids in the juice, and lignans in the toast).

Eat your fruits and vegetables. A recent study by Penn State researchers shows that eating more fruits and vegetables (at least four and a half cups per day) could help to prevent weight gain—even when your overall diet is high in fat. About 90 percent of Americans do not eat enough fruits and vegetables—and over ninety million of us suffer chronic diseases as a result. Go figure—the most popular "vegetable" in the country is the French fry, and of the limited produce that we do eat, 40 percent comes from potatoes, corn, and peas (according to the Centers for Disease Control). The Institute of Medicine, the Department of Agriculture, and the Department of Health and Human Services all want us to eat more fruits and veggies because scientific research shows us that "more is better" in terms of reducing the risk for obesity, diabetes, osteoporosis, stroke, heart disease, and many cancers. A forty-year-old woman, for example, should eat two and a half cups of vegetables and one and a half cups of fruit daily, while a sixty-five-year-old man should eat the same amount of vegetables and fruit plus an additional half cup of fruit. (The now out-of-date "five-a-day" recommendations called for only about two and a half cups of fruits and vegetables.)

When choosing your fruits and vegetables, any are better than none, but those that are darker colored (dark green, dark blue/purple, bright orange, bright red, bright yellow, etc.) tend to be better sources of vitamins, minerals, and phytonutrients. According to researchers at the University of Washington, the "best" fruits in terms of nutrient content and disease prevention include cantaloupe, tangerines, blueberries, apricots, and raspberries, while the "best" vegetables include spinach, romaine lettuce, broccoli, tomatoes, and bell peppers.

Phytonutrients are specialized vitamin-like compounds found in plants (*phyto-* means *plant*) that provide numerous health benefits. In general, the brighter in color the fruit or vegetable, the higher the content of particular phytonutrients. For example, lycopene, a red carotenoid, is found at high levels in tomatoes, while another carotenoid, beta-carotene, is responsible for the orange color of carrots and sweet potatoes. A simple (and fun) way to maximize your intake of phytonutrients and other micronutrients is to "color" your diet by trying to eat as many different colored fruits and vegetables as possible. Try shooting for five different colors each day: one serving each that is red (tomato), blue or purple (berries), yellow (melon), orange (carrot), and green (broccoli)—or whatever colors you can find. (Note: French fries do not count as a yellow vegetable.)

In terms of the macronutrients, many dieticians and nutritionists forget the concept of balance by guiding their clients toward a diet high in complex carbohydrates. While it is perfectly acceptable for most of us to focus our diet on increasing the amount of complex carbohydrates we eat, we must not forget to balance those carbohydrates with proper amounts of protein, fat, and fiber. During anxious or highly stressful times, we may even crave carbohydrates such as bread and sweets. Part of this is due to the effect of cortisol to suppress insulin function, increase blood-sugar levels, and stimulate appetite. In addition, however, your brain may urge you to eat more carbohydrates because they can act as a "tranquilizer" of sorts by increasing brain levels of serotonin (the neurotransmitter that calms us down). Unfortunately, while caving into the urges and chowing down on the carbs may give you a euphoric feeling for a few minutes, you'll surely pay for it later in the form of low energy levels, mood swings, more cravings, and a tendency toward weight gain.

Then there's the opposite problem. Some popular dietary advice takes the view that proteins are "good" and carbohydrates are "bad." Following such misguided instruction leads people to consume too much protein and not enough carbohydrate, again missing the point that what they should be striving for is the right balance of each. Achieving the right balance is of key importance, because each of the macronutrients performs a different primary role in the body. Protein can be thought of as the primary tissue builder (and rebuilder) because it helps us to maintain lean muscle mass. On the other hand, consuming more protein than a person needs, as one might do when using some of the very high protein bodybuilding drink mixes, can lead to dehydration and bloating. Carbohydrate consumption is vital because it serves as the primary fuel for the brain (which cannot use any other fuel source as efficiently), as well as a metabolic enhancer to encourage the body to use fat as a fuel source. A popular saying among metabolic physiologists is "fat burns in the flame of carbohydrate," which means that the breakdown products of carbohydrate metabolism are required for the optimal breakdown of stored body fat and the conversion of that fat into energy. Finally, both fat and fiber are needed to round out the balanced macronutrient mix because they both work to slow digestion and absorption of carbohydrates, control blood-sugar levels, and induce satiety (feelings of fullness). Additionally, certain kinds of dietary fat provide our only sources of the essential fatty acids (EFAs), linoleic acid and linolenic acid. These have been shown to help lower cholesterol and blood pressure, reduce the risk of heart disease, stroke, and possibly some kinds of cancer, and prevent dry hair and skin.

Protein Needs

That's all well and good: We need to have *some* carbohydrate and *some* protein at every meal—but how much? Let's start with our protein requirements. Very good research over the past decade or so shows that people who do a moderate amount of regular exercise (which you should be doing anyway for its cortisol-control benefits) need between 1.2 and 1.8 grams of protein per kilogram of body weight per day. You don't need to worry about all the mathematical gibberish, but you do need to understand that this means that a smaller person will need less protein in a given day than a larger person, simply because the larger person has more mass to support. For a 140-pound person, the math works out to about 77–115 grams of protein per day (let's say the average is 100 grams). For a 200-pound person, the protein requirement works out to 110–165 grams per day (we'll average that to 140 grams). Now, assuming that you're eating five to six small meals/snacks per day (as you should for optimal energy levels, appetite control, and fat metabolism), this amount of protein breaks down to about 20 grams per meal for the 140-pound person and not quite 30 grams per meal for the 200-pound person. Remember that eating more protein than this at each meal will not do anything extra in terms of muscle building; it will just add calories to your diet and increase your risk of becoming dehydrated and having gas.

Carbohydrate Needs

The next piece of the puzzle—the amount of carbohydrate you need—is determined largely by your weight-loss needs and your exercise patterns. If you need to lose weight, then you'll want to stay toward the low end of the recommended range (but avoid going too much lower, because fat metabolism will suffer). If you find yourself doing more than thirty minutes of exercise each day, then you'll want to be toward the high end of the recommended range (but not too much above it because of problems with insulin, blood-sugar control, and weight gain). So how much? First of all, let's realize that your brain wants to use carbohydrates (and carbohydrates only) for its energy needs. This amount generally works out to be about 100 grams of carbohydrate per day; without that amount, brain function slows down, you feel less "sharp," and your ability to concentrate is compromised. So you need at least 100 grams of carbohydrate (balanced with protein) in your daily diet. Do you need more? If you are also exercising (which you should be), then you'll need another 200–250 grams to support the needs of your muscles during intense efforts. Keeping in mind that "fat burns in the flame of carbohydrate" and that you should be eating five to six meals/snacks per day, then the math works out to about 50–60 grams of carbohydrate per meal.

Putting all of the above mumbo jumbo together will have you consuming five to six meals/snacks per day, each one composed of 20–30 grams of protein plus 50–60 grams of carbohydrate, which works out to a total caloric level of 280–360 calories per meal. If you then add to each meal/snack 3–5 grams of fiber (which contains no calories) and 3–5 grams of fat (30–45 additional calories) and you get optimal blood-sugar control, appetite regulation, enhanced fat metabolism, increased energy levels, better mood, and many more benefits. (Also, check out the "Nutrition" section in Chapter 9, which provides tools for gauging appropriate serving sizes to meet these requirements.)

> *Becky,* like millions of people, was constantly fighting a losing battle against her weight and her hunger—especially in the late afternoon and early evening when she was most likely to crave a sweet snack. When her stress went up, so did her eating and her body weight. Unfortunately, although she was committed

to doing what she thought to be the "right" things for weight loss, by skipping breakfast and following an extremely low-fat diet for the rest of the day she was using the wrong weapons in her battle of the bulge.

Becky's solution was to completely revamp her dietary regimen so that she ate something every three to four hours throughout the day. That "something"—whether it was a meal or a snack—was balanced to provide moderate amounts of carbohydrate and protein to help control blood sugar and regulate appetite. The immediate benefits for Becky were a dramatic decrease in her afternoon and evening cravings, an easier time sticking to her diet, and a ten-pound loss of body fat within two months.

SUPPLEMENTS

With all this emphasis on getting enough sleep, doing some exercise, and eating the right amounts of macronutrients and micronutrients, where do dietary supplements fit in? Aside from avoiding the herbal stimulants mentioned above (which can *increase* cortisol levels), a variety of dietary supplements exist that can help control the hypersecretion of cortisol, keeping it within optimal ranges even when a person is under stress.

Whether one's exposure to stress is the result of physical or psychological factors, the response mounted by the body's hormonal system is exactly the same (and is equally detrimental). This means physical stressors such as suboptimal nutrition (dieting), extremes of exercise, or inadequate sleep will affect the body in many of the same ways as psychological stressors such as concerns about body image, worry, and anger. No matter what source of stress a person is exposed to, the body proceeds through a systemic stress response that increases levels of cortisol and leads to many of the associated declines in health. However, advances in nutritional science have shown that a wide variety of dietary and herbal ingredients can instead assist the body in mounting an *adaptive* response to stress and help to minimize or control some of these systemic effects of stress. These natural products represent a logical and convenient approach for many people who are subjected to stressors on a daily basis; for example, from work, finances, and/or the environment. For most of us most of the time, *removing* the stressor (avoiding it) is an impossible option, no matter how desirable that option may be. Think about it: We all have to work (stress!), we all have to pay our bills on time (stress!), many of us have to sit in rush-hour traffic (stress!), and we all have family and interpersonal relationships that don't always go smoothly (stress!). Most of us also know that we *should* be eating better and that we *should* be getting more exercise (both of which can help control the stress response)—but the reality of our busy lives means that other things often take priority over exercise (job, kids, spouse, chores, you name it). In addition, the very concept of taking time out of these busy schedules for a yoga or meditation class is downright laughable, even though we know it would likely do us a lot of good.

For many, the only logical solution to managing an overactive stress response may be the use of certain dietary supplements to help control the body's excessive exposure to cortisol. By keeping cortisol levels within an optimal range, many of the potential adverse effects of acute and chronic stress can be held at bay—and taking the right combination of dietary supplements can be a safe, effective, and convenient approach for doing so.

As of this writing, the most promising cortisol-control supplements include the following (each of which is covered in more detail in Chapter 8):

Vitamins and Minerals for Stress Adaptation

Daily use of the following is recommended for everybody, from Stressed Jess to Strained Jane to Relaxed Jack:

- B-complex vitamins
- Vitamin C
- Magnesium
- Calcium

Supplements for Targeted Cortisol Control

Daily use of the following supplements is recommended for Stressed Jess and Strained Jane, but Relaxed Jack needs these supplements only during periods of especially high stress:

- Magnolia bark
- Theanine
- Phytosterols
- PMFs (polymethoxylated flavones; for more on these, see Chapter 8)
- Eurycoma

Support Supplements for Use During Heightened Stress

Occasional use of the following supplements is recommended for Stressed Jess and Strained Jane only when they need additional help relaxing or sleeping. Relaxed Jack generally has no additional need for supplements beyond those for targeted cortisol control.

- Ashwagandha
- Ginseng
- Schisandra
- Rhodiola
- Kava kava
- Valerian
- St. John's wort
- 5-HTP (5-hydroxytryptophan; for more on this, see Chapter 8)
- SAM-e (S-adenosylmethionine; for more on this, see Chapter 8)

The next chapter focuses on helping you personalize a supplement program for your own specific needs. But first, how does one go about choosing and using dietary supplements? Where should you shop for supplements, and how do you select the best brand? Should you use supplements if you're taking prescription medications? Can supplements make up for an inadequate diet?

These are all good questions, and the following section answers them—and more.

GUIDELINES FOR CHOOSING AND USING DIETARY SUPPLEMENTS

Without a doubt, dietary supplements have widespread usage and appeal, to the tune of more than $22 billion in annual sales in the United States alone. Approximately 85 percent of Americans have used dietary supplements at one time or another, and more than 60 percent of the population are regular users of supplements (using them on most days of the week).

Despite the large number of people currently buying and using dietary supplements, a huge gap often exists between the practice of supplementation and the knowledge behind these choices and usage patterns. For example, while virtually 100 percent of adults consult their doctors or pharmacists about how to use prescriptions, less than half discuss dietary supplements with a health-care professional. In addition, many consumers are not careful about recommended dosages for supplements—and the common assumption that "if one is good, more is better" can pose serious health consequences for some supplement users.

It is very important that you discuss your use of dietary supplements with your health-care provider. In many cases that health professional will not be an expert in nutrition or supplementation, but the knowledge that you are supplementing your diet will at least alert your health-care provider to issues such as the possibility for drug interactions or blood thinning.

It is also important that supplements be used responsibly. Just because they're not prescription drugs, it is dangerous to think that they can be used indiscriminately. Chapter 8 of this book can be used as a sort of handbook for supplements that target cortisol control, and the case studies presented throughout the book can help you decide on the most appropriate use of these supplements for your particular situation. For supplement recommendations in areas other than cortisol control, a consultation with a qualified nutritionist, dietician, herbalist, or nutritionally oriented physician is appropriate. Rather than blindly picking a consultant out of the yellow pages, you can check with the following organizations to find a qualified supplement consultant in your area:

American Nutraceutical Association (www.america
nutra.com)

American College of Nutrition (www.am-coll-nutr.org)

American Dietetic Association (www.eatright.org)

SupplementWatch, Inc. (www.supplementwatch.com)

However, for some of the more straightforward supplement questions and answers, the following information can help guide you in choosing and using the right supplements in the proper manner.

CHOOSING SUPPLEMENTS

Below, I've answered some of the most common questions about how to choose among the many supplements available.

Q: Are natural forms of vitamins better than synthetic forms?

A: In most cases, natural and synthetic vitamins and minerals are handled by the body in exactly the same way. A good example of this is the B-complex vitamins, which can be obtained in supplements as "natural" B vitamins (usually from brewer's yeast or a similar substance) or as purified chemicals that are listed on the product label as thiamin (B-1), riboflavin (B-2), niacin (B-3), and so forth. When either of these supplemental sources of B vitamins is consumed, the vitamins are absorbed, transported, and utilized by the body in exactly the same way—so we can say with confidence that there is no difference between natural and synthetic when it comes to B vitamins. Two interesting exceptions to this example are folic acid, which is better absorbed as the synthetic form (compared to natural forms found in foods), and vitamin E, which is far superior in the natural versus the synthetic form. In the case of vitamin E, very good scientific data exist showing that natural vitamin E is absorbed and retained in the body two to three times better than the synthetic forms. Natural vitamin E costs a bit more than the synthetic variety, but the small added cost is more than justified by the higher activity.

Q: **Should I choose a brand-name or generic vitamin/mineral supplement?**

A: The ultimate answer to this question is less about generics or brand-name products than it is about choosing between supplements that provide "basic" versus "optimal" levels of particular nutrients. Therefore, your answer to this question will depend on two primary factors: How much money can you afford to spend on a supplement, and are you looking for a basic or an optimal supplement?

Many of the generic or private-label store-brand supplements on the market will do a satisfactory job of helping you meet the basic RDA (recommended daily allowance) levels for essential vitamins and minerals. The primary limitation with these generic products, and even with many brand-name supplements, is that the basic RDA levels of most vitamins and minerals fall far below the levels associated with optimal health and certainly below those needed for optimal cortisol control. Chapter 8 outlines many of the details surrounding the use of vitamins and minerals for cortisol control, but a couple of the most important are worth highlighting here:

With respect to the B vitamins, there is very good scientific evidence to support daily intakes at 200–500 percent of RDA levels for optimal stress response and cortisol control. These levels are two to five times higher than the levels found in most multivitamin products.

Calcium and magnesium are two minerals that are known to help regulate the body's stress response, yet most generic supplements and "one-tablet-a-day" type brand-name supplements provide only a small fraction of the 250–500 milligrams (mg) of calcium and the 125–250 mg of magnesium needed to aid cortisol control. The primary reason for skimping on the calcium and magnesium in these products is due not to costs (both are very cheap), but to space considerations in the capsules and tablets. Both calcium and magnesium are bulky minerals—that is, they take up a lot of space—so an optimal daily dosage requires more than a single capsule each day (and sometimes as many as four capsules, depending on the mineral source).

The bottom line here is that everybody should take at least a basic multivitamin/multimineral supplement—and virtually any product, generic or brand-name, found on the shelf at Wal-Mart, Rite-Aid, or your local grocery store will satisfy the basic RDA-level requirements. However, if you are interested in a supplement that delivers more than the rock-bottom levels of cortisol-controlling nutrients, and if you can afford to spend a little more on your daily supplement regimen, then you will want to consider a multivitamin/mineral supplement that provides higher levels of B-complex vitamins, calcium, and magnesium.

Q: **What should I consider when I am shopping for herbal supplements?**

A: When it comes to selecting herbal supplements, the situation can quickly get very confusing. Because herbals are really a form of natural medicine, it is crucial that you select the right form of the herb so that you get the safest and most effective product. Herbal supplements are absolutely an area in which generic products are *not* equivalent to brand-name products. It is vitally important to select either the exact product that has been used in clinical studies, or a product that contains a chemically equivalent form of the herb that has been studied. The easiest way for most consumers to select a safe and effective herb is to select only those extracts that have been "standardized" in order to provide a uniform level of the key active ingredients in each batch of the product (see the supplement descriptions in Chapter 8 for details on these standards). The best scenario would be to select only those specific *products* that have undergone clinical studies of their own (rather than selecting products that contain *ingredients* on which studies have been conducted)—but there are far fewer finished products that have been subjected to clinical testing than there are raw ingredients (magnolia bark, theanine, etc.) that have been evaluated in such research.

Q: Where is the best place to buy supplements?
A: The preceding three responses should you offer enough general guidance to help you weed through the many less desirable supplement products on the market and select products that can make a difference in your overall health. With the explosive growth in the supplement market over the past decade, consumers can now find vitamins, minerals, herbs, and other supplements for sale in a variety of places—including specialty supplement stores, natural-foods stores, grocery stores, drugstores, discount department stores, and through direct marketing, infomercials, catalog sales, and the Internet. Is any one of these outlets better than the others? Not really—but they each have their own particular niche.

For example, the least expensive "bargain" products will be found at supermarkets and discount department stores (e.g., Wal-Mart), but these products may suffer from many of the problems outlined above with regard to basic versus optimal supplementation. Supplements that are a step above the cheapest and most basic of products can typically be found at drugstores, natural-foods markets, and specialty supplement outlets.

These are the middle-of-the-road products that do a decent job of balancing high-quality and optimal nutrient levels with moderate prices.

The most expensive products, and those with the widest range in terms of quality, safety, and effectiveness, are typically sold through direct sales channels such as the Internet, catalogs, and independent sales agents. In some cases, these products are designed to deliver optimal levels of all nutrients in the most bioavailable forms, but the obvious downside is their high price. In other cases, all you get is the high price—without any of the optimal levels of the crucial nutrients. So how can you differentiate between these premium-priced products? By asking to see the results from their clinical studies. Products in this "premium" category will almost certainly need to justify their high price with strong scientific evidence to support their claims and to show that their product is justified at this price. If the company cannot provide you with scientific evidence to support its premium products, then you are well advised to look elsewhere for your supplement.

USING SUPPLEMENTS

After you have selected your supplements with the help of the above information, the following guidelines can help you to use those supplements in the proper manner (that is, so you optimize both safety and effectiveness):

- Remember that a dietary supplement is just that—meaning that it is meant to be *added to* an otherwise healthy diet. It is not meant to substitute for a balanced diet or to make up for a poor diet.

- Follow the dosage recommendations on the package. The recommended dosage is important for safety and effectiveness—especially for herbals and other supplements that combine multiple ingredients. Don't make the mistaken assumption that if one tablet is recommended per day, two or three will be even better.

- Keep all dietary supplements in a safe place—away from heat and light that may accelerate their breakdown, and away from children who may accidentally ingest them.

- Talk to your health-care provider about any dietary supplements you are taking. If you are on any form of prescription or over-the-counter medication, talk with your doctor or pharmacist *before* using *any* supplements.

CHAPTER 8

Dietary Supplements
for Stress Adaptation

Y ou'll notice that supplements are the *fourth* part of the overall SENSE program—coming *after* stress management, exercise, and nutrition. I firmly believe, and the research strongly
supports, that adding a targeted supplement regimen to your overall program will enhance your benefits in terms of stress reduction,
cortisol control, and well-being.

Keep in mind that my supplement recommendations are not,
and never have been, anything along the "take a pill and you'll be
fine" line of thinking that you'll undoubtedly encounter among the
many miracle weight-loss products that are on the market. Again,
the role of a supplement is just that—to *supplement* a healthy diet
and exercise regimen.

SUPPLEMENTS VERSUS
PRESCRIPTION DRUGS

Are supplements safe? For the most part, yes. I say, "for the most
part" to emphasize the importance of taking supplements only as
they are recommended to be used. The vast majority of problems
associated with dietary supplements result from improper use—
such as taking too much in an attempt to get a "faster" or "greater"

effect. It is not uncommon to find people taking a double or triple dose of a particular supplement because they want to lose weight faster. DO NOT fall for the myth of "more is better" when it comes to supplements, because more often than not, more ends up being *worse* in terms of safety and effectiveness. Instead, follow the dosage guidelines listed on every supplement you are taking—and discontinue immediately if you experience any adverse side effects.

When we compare the safety profiles of natural supplements to those of synthetic drugs, the differences are striking. There are currently over three million adverse event reports (AERs) in the FDA's MedWatch database for drugs, but there are very few for dietary supplements. In the last ten years, during which several billion supplement doses have been consumed in this country, we're talking about possibly a few hundred AERs for supplements—almost all of which were due to improper use of the supplement, such as taking more than the label recommends. As far as safety profiles go, it is hard to beat the safety record for dietary supplements.

One of the reasons for the superior safety profile of supplements compared to drugs is that supplements are less potent—and a lower potency generally means fewer side effects. Even at this reduced potency, supplements may actually be just as effective as a more potent drug for producing certain positive outcomes. Because natural supplements often have dozens or even hundreds of different constituents, they can work on several aspects of metabolism simultaneously. For example, an antidepressant like Prozac may have a very potent effect on a single neurotransmitter in the brain (serotonin), while a natural supplement such as St. John's wort may help to modulate and balance several different neurotransmitters at the same time. This "multifunction" effect of natural supplements, versus the "single-effect" of synthetic drugs, has the potential to both increase effectiveness and decrease side effects.

How many drugs do we have for treating stress and the "metabolism of stress"? None! Instead, doctors will often prescribe antidepressants for stress-related mood problems and appetite suppressants for stress-induced eating—but none of these drugs addresses the root problem (and, thus, they are only marginally effective for most people). Consider the most popular drugs for "treating" obesity: Rimonabant/Acomplia, which causes side effects such as depression and anxiety; Sibutramine/Meridia, which causes side effects such as high blood pressure and anxiety; and Orlistat/Xenical, which causes side effects such as gastrointestinal problems. Each of these drugs delivers only an additional five to ten extra pounds of weight loss per year (when added to a diet/exercise regimen)—and they only work for about 50 percent of the people who try them! If that weren't a poor cost/benefit relationship, consider the fact that these drugs cost $100–$150 per month (or about $200 per pound of weight that you *might* lose)! The various side effects come with no extra charge.

Given the *huge* profit potential for drugs to treat stress-related conditions such as obesity, depression, diabetes, and fatigue, the "off-label" use of many drugs is growing—especially among those trying to lose weight. Drugs approved for treating diabetes, depression, and epilepsy are increasingly used by dieters because of their weight-loss side effects. None of these drugs has been studied or approved for safe weight loss, but because weight loss is a side effect of their main effect, some patients are asking their doctors (and the doctors are agreeing) to prescribe these drugs for weight loss. Among the growing list are drugs meant to treat attention-deficit hyperactivity disorder (Adderall and Ritalin), epilepsy (Topamax and Zonegran), depression (Wellbutrin), diabetes (Glucophage and Byetta), sleep disorders (Provigil), and smoking (Zyban).

Often, these drugs are used alone, but sometimes they're used in combinations that were never intended, or certainly not recommended, when they were allowed on the market. For example, Adderall is a stimulant that was originally marketed as a diet drug in the 1970s and has now become the weight-loss agent of choice among folks ranging from Hollywood starlets to soccer moms (most of whom take it without a prescription for the ADHD it is intended to treat).

Aside from the annoying side effects that many of these drugs carry, such as abdominal cramps, anxiety, insomnia, and memory problems, some of the drugs (such as Wellbutrin) carry the FDA's harshest "black box" warning, informing consumers about an increased risk of suicide. Adderall also carries a black box warning because it can cause sudden death, serious cardiovascular events, and addiction. Topamax causes confusion and mental disturbances, and Provigil leads to dizziness and insomnia in many people.

Used alone or in combination, monthly costs for most of these drugs easily run close to $200. Typical drug cocktails might consist of Phentermine (a stimulant) plus the antidepressant Prozac, anti-seizure drugs like Topamax, or diabetes drugs such as Byetta. Often, patients are told that because obesity is a chronic disease, they will need to take these drugs for life—or until the side effects are no longer tolerable.

As clear evidence that these drugs are being used "off label" for weight loss, sales of Adderall XR (a stimulant) increased more than 3,000 percent between 2001 and 2005, while sales of Provigil (also a stimulant) increased more than 360 percent. Last year, sales of Wellbutrin XL (a once-daily depression drug) were up more than 1,000 percent, to $1.4 billion in sales. At the same time, sales of the only two FDA-approved obesity drugs (Orlistat and Meridia) were down more than 40 percent, because they don't work very well for weight loss.

Given the high cost of drugs, in terms of both money and side effects, it is logical to look to natural options to control stress, manage cortisol exposure, and modulate the biochemical stress response. The sections that follow outline some of the most effective natural supplements for adapting to stress, including:

- "Stress-formula" vitamin/mineral supplements
- Cortisol-control supplements
- HSD-balancing supplements
- Testosterone-control supplements
- Adaptogens
- Relaxation and calming supplements

But first, let's review which supplements to steer clear of.

SUPPLEMENTS TO AVOID

As indicated in previous chapters, high cortisol levels are associated with being overweight, and yet at the same time cortisol levels
are elevated by dieting and by cognitive dietary restraint (a fancy
term for thinking about dieting). It is no wonder, then, that people
who are under chronic or repeated stress tend to struggle with their
weight, their appetite, and their energy levels—all of which are im-
pacted by the elevated cortisol levels associated with their stress.
It would seem to be a virtual miracle for a dietary supplement to
come along with claims of increasing weight loss, suppressing appetite, and boosting energy levels. In fact, this supplement would
almost seem to be tailor-made for people under stress, because it
addresses three of the key factors that lead them down the path to
weight gain.

The "miracle" supplements described above fall into a category
of herbal stimulants that function as *sympathomimetics*—meaning
they mimic some of the effects of the body's own sympathetic
(stimulant) hormones such as epinephrine and norepinephrine,
either by increasing the secretion of those hormones or by reducing their breakdown. Among the most popular herbals in this category are *Ephedra sinensis* (ma huang), *Paullinia cupana* (guarana/
caffeine), *Citrus aurantium* (synephrine), *Pausinystalia yohimbe* (yohimbine), and *Coleus forskohlii* (forskolin)—but many other plant
species contain related stimulant compounds. Each of these herbs
acts as a general stimulant on many parts of the body simultaneously, including the lungs (where they can open bronchioles to
make breathing easier), the heart and blood vessels (where they increase heart rate and constrict arteries to increase blood pressure),
and even the adrenal glands (where they stimulate the secretion of
epinephrine and cortisol). Because of these wide-ranging actions in
many tissues, the herbal stimulants are also frequently associated
with a number of adverse side effects such as headaches, insomnia, elevated blood pressure, irritability, and heart palpitations. But
perhaps the side effect that provokes the most concern is the large
increase in cortisol levels caused by these substances.

The widespread popularity of the herbal stimulants—most no-tably ephedra—is due largely to the fact that they work (at least in the short-term). Ephedra and related supplements are well known to kill appetite and increase energy levels, so you either exercise more or you fidget more, but either way you burn some extra calo-ries. This means that over the course of a month or two, the herbal stimulant products will help a person drop a few more pounds than he otherwise would have been able to do on his own. The down-side, however, is the fact that while the short-term effects of these compounds are beneficial for weight loss (by reducing appetite and increasing caloric expenditure), the longer-term increase in corti-sol levels is detrimental for weight-loss efforts. Why? Because, as outlined previously, the increase in cortisol levels will increase hun-ger, slow down fat metabolism, eat away at muscles and bones, sap energy, wreck mood, and generally thwart attempts to maintain a healthy body weight.

So here we have a class of weight-loss supplements that pro-vides some actual benefits when used for a few weeks, but then turns on the user to cause a series of metabolic changes in the body that *promote* weight gain over several months. If that news isn't already bad enough, it also appears that the tendency of ephedra and related compounds to cause weight gain over a longer period of time is even stronger when the user is experiencing an additional stressor (and dieting is a stressor). Researchers from Lausanne Uni-versity, in Switzerland, found that as little as two days of ephedra consumption, at 40 milligrams (mg) per day, reduced glucose up-take and oxidation by 25 percent. When subjects were under ad-ditional stress, the fall in glucose uptake and oxidation exceeded 50 percent! This means ephedra supplements inhibit the body's abil-ity to use glucose as an energy source, so blood-sugar levels climb, fat metabolism shuts off, and hunger comes raging back. Similar findings have been noted for forskolin (the active ingredient in *Coleus forskohlii*), yohimbine (the active ingredient in *Pausinystalia yohimbe*), and caffeine (the active ingredient in yerba mate, Kola nut, and *Paullinia cupana*, also known as guarana). For example, approximately 200 mg of caffeine (about the amount contained in two cups of coffee and in a single dose of many weight-loss supplements) will increase blood levels of cortisol by 30 percent within one hour. Researchers from the University of Oklahoma have shown that caffeine not only causes elevations in cortisol levels, but also that the combination of caffeine intake plus increased stress causes an even bigger jump in cortisol exposure (and when do we drink the most coffee? Yep, when we're under stress). The Oklahoma scientists found that both men and women respond to caffeine plus stress with much higher cortisol levels—and that repeated doses of caffeine continue to increase cortisol levels throughout the day.

What we see in the longer-term studies of herbal stimulants is a persistent elevation in plasma cortisol levels caused by a stresslike neuroendocrine response to stimulation of the brain and the adrenal glands. In animal studies, this type of nervous-system stimulation leads not only to elevated cortisol levels, but also to reductions in levels of growth hormone and thyroid-stimulating hormone, both of which are involved in keeping us lean.

So what to do? The most prudent approach would be to completely avoid these herbal stimulants in favor of a more balanced approach to promoting weight loss, such as eating several small meals spaced throughout the day, consuming a balanced intake of protein/carbs/fat/fiber, and getting regular aerobic exercise (plus resistance training). That said, millions of people are likely to keep using products that have herbal stimulants in them. Despite the long-term risk to overall health and the sabotage such supplements can inflict on a person's weight-maintenance efforts, the quick-fix promise of dropping a few extra pounds in a few weeks is simply too much for many people to resist. If you *do* decide to use any of these herbal stimulants, please do so with extreme caution—and try to curb your use of them after one month. At the very least, the cortisol-*raising* effects of the herbal stimulants should be counteracted by combining their use with one of the cortisol-lowering herbs outlined later in this chapter. It is unlikely that the cortisol-controlling supplements will counteract either the appetite-control or the thermogenic/fat-burning effects of the herbal stimulants, but they will certainly lessen the adverse side effects of elevated cortisol.

The rest of this section provides brief summaries of each of the most popular herbal stimulants used in weight-loss supplements.

Ma Huang/Ephedra

Ma huang is a Chinese herb that is also referred to as *Chinese ephedra (Ephedra sinensis)* and *herbal ephedrine.* The active compounds—ephedra or ephedrine alkaloids—are also found in other herbals, such as Mormon tea and *Sida cordifolia,* and may be referred to by common names such as desert tea, Mexican tea, sea grape, and many others. Overall, about forty species of plants contain versions of ephedra.

Ma huang and its various herbal cousins function as sympathomimetics, the effects of which are described earlier in this chapter. Ephedrine is considered a *nonselective sympathomimetic,* which means that it acts as a general stimulant on many parts of the body simultaneously (lungs, heart, blood vessels, adrenal glands, and others). Therefore, it can give users a boost or pickup similar to what they might feel after a cup or two of strong coffee. By mimicking the effects of epinephrine, ephedra can increase the output of blood from the heart, enhance muscle contractility, raise blood-sugar levels, and open bronchial pathways for easier breathing. In many cases, ephedra can result in a temporary suppression of appetite, which may help efforts aimed at dietary restriction and weight loss.

The research findings concerning the effects of ma huang and other ephedra-containing products are equivocal; some studies do not show any beneficial effect, some studies show a modest increase in weight loss, and still other studies become unreliable, due to high numbers of subjects dropping out due to unpleasant side effects. Because ephedrine is a stimulant, it is logical that either a single dose or chronic repeated use would elevate metabolic rate somewhat (meaning the user would burn more calories at rest and during exercise). Various studies of overweight men and women have shown that the combination of ephedrine (20–40 mg) and caffeine (200–400 mg) produces a slight increase in resting metabolism.

The Food and Drug Administration (FDA) has received more than a thousand reports of adverse side effects from consumers who have used supplements containing ephedrine alkaloids. Complaints have ranged from nervous-system and cardiovascular-system effects, such as elevated blood pressure and heart palpitations, to insomnia, irritability, headaches, and more serious adverse effects, such as seizures, stroke, heart attack, and even death (about fifteen to twenty thus far). Most of these adverse events occurred in otherwise healthy, young to middle-aged adults who were using the products for weight control or increased energy.

Health Warning for Ephedra-Containing Dietary Supplements

Virtually all dietary supplements that contain ephedra alkaloids also carry a strong warning on their label. It reads something like the following:

Women who are pregnant or nursing should avoid using ephedra-containing products. Keep out of reach of children. Avoid using ephedrine-containing products if you have high blood pressure, heart or thyroid disease, diabetes, difficulty in urination due to prostate enlargement, or if taking monoamine oxidase (MAO) inhibitors or any other prescription drug. Reduce or discontinue use if nervousness, tremor, irritability, rapid heartbeat, sleeplessness, loss of appetite, or nausea occurs.

Across the full range of studies that have been conducted on products containing ephedra for weight loss, the total amount of ephedrine ingested per day has ranged from 60 to 75 mg of ephedrine alone (usually in three doses of 20–25 mg each) to 20–40 mg of ephedrine combined with 200–400 mg of caffeine. It is important to note, however, that these dosage recommendations should be considered in light of recent studies showing that the levels of ephedra alkaloids can vary by as much as 1,000 percent from one dietary supplement to another.

The purified versions of ephedra (ephedrine and pseudoephedrine) found in many over-the-counter cold medicines have the very same effect on cortisol levels (raising them). However, in contrast to ephedra-based weight-loss supplements, which might be used for many weeks at a time (and thus lead to chronically high cortisol levels), typical cold remedies are used for no more than a few days in a row and thus would cause only a temporary rise in cortisol levels.

Should you decide to use ephedra-containing products, it is important to understand that while the *short-term* effects (suppressed appetite and slight increase in caloric expenditure) might give your weight-loss efforts a boost, the *longer-term* effects (chronically elevated cortisol levels) will sabotage your ability to maintain that weight loss. Therefore, ephedra supplements should be used for no more than six to twelve weeks, and even then, for optimal effect, they should be balanced with supplements that help to control cortisol levels.

Guarana

Guarana *(Paullinia cupana)* comes from the seeds of a Brazilian plant. Traditional uses of guarana by natives of the Amazonian rain forest include adding crushed seeds of the plant to foods and beverages to increase alertness and reduce fatigue. As a dietary supplement, it's no wonder guarana is an effective energy booster; it contains approximately twice the caffeine found in coffee beans. Guarana seeds are about 3–4 percent caffeine, compared to the 1–2 percent in coffee beans. Concentrated guarana extracts, however, can contain as much as 40–50 percent caffeine, with popular supplements delivering 50–200 mg of caffeine per day, about the same amount found in one or two cups of strong coffee. Guarana is generally considered to be as safe for healthy people as caffeine. As with any caffeine-containing substance, guarana extracts can lead to insomnia, nervousness, anxiety, headaches, high blood pressure, and heart palpitations.

The theory behind how guarana works is relatively straightforward. The major active constituents are caffeine (sometimes called *guaranine* to make the user think it is different in some way) and similar alkaloids such as theobromine and theophylline, which are also found in coffee and tea. Each of these compounds has well-known effects as nervous-system stimulants. As such, they may also bear some effect on increasing metabolic rate, suppressing appetite, and enhancing both physical and mental performance.

Most of the scientific evidence on caffeine as a general stimulant and an aid to exercise performance shows convincingly that caffeine is effective. As a weight-loss aid, however, although high doses of caffeine may somewhat suppress appetite, on its own it does not seem to be a very effective supplement for increasing caloric expenditure (thermogenesis). However, when combined with other stimulant-type supplements, such as ma huang (ephedra), it appears that caffeine can extend the duration of ephedra's action in suppressing appetite and increasing caloric expenditure; it is unknown whether caffeine may also increase the risk of adverse side effects.

Synephrine

Synephrine is the main active compound found in the fruit of a plant called *Citrus aurantium*. The fruit is also known as *zhi shi* in traditional Chinese medicine, and as *green orange, sour orange,* and *bitter orange* in other parts of the world. Synephrine is chemically very similar to the ephedrine found in a number of weight-loss and energy supplements that contain ma huang. But synephrine differs from ephedrine in that synephrine is considered a *semiselective sympathomimetic* (because it targets some tissues, such as fat, more than it targets others, such as the heart) versus a *nonselective sympathomimetic* (like ephedra, which targets many tissues equally and thus often causes side effects). For example, although some high-dose ephedra-containing supplements have been associated with certain cardiovascular side effects such as elevated blood pressure and heart palpitations, researchers at Mercer University, in Atlanta, have shown that *Citrus aurantium* extract has no effect on hemodynamics such as heart rate and blood pressure because it targets fat tissue rather than heart tissue.

Because synephrine, like caffeine and ephedrine, is a mild stimulant, it is also thought to have similar effects in terms of providing an energy boost, suppressing appetite, and increasing metabolic rate and caloric expenditure. In traditional Chinese medicine, zhi shi is used to help stimulate *qi* (pronounced *chee,* and defined as the body's vital energy or life force), but in order to maximize the metabolic benefits of these extracts, total synephrine intake should probably be kept to a range of 2–10 mg per day.

One study in dogs suggests that the synephrine and octopamine found in *Citrus aurantium* extracts can increase metabolic rate in a specific type of fat tissue known as brown adipose tissue (BAT). This effect would be expected to increase fat loss in humans, except for one small detail: Adult humans don't have any brown adipose tissue to speak of. Despite this fact, this claim still stands as one of the most overhyped promises on the weight-loss scene. Since being introduced to the marketplace more than 10 years ago, synephrine-containing supplements have existed solely because of some interesting theories on how they *might* work to increase metabolic rate and promote significant weight loss. At this writing, there is still a glaring lack of credible research showing any weight loss effects of synephrine-containing supplements in humans. In fact, most of the available human clinical trials on synephrine-based supplements suggest that the supplements are not particularly effective for promoting weight loss.

Yohimbe

Yohimbe (*Pausinystalia yohimbe*) comes from the bark of an African tree; the active compound, an alkaloid called yohimbine, can also be found in high amounts in the South American herb quebracho (*Aspidosperma quebracho-blanco*). It has traditionally been used as a stimulant and aphrodisiac in both West Africa and South America. In the United States, yohimbe and quebracho are most often promoted in dietary supplements for treating impotence, stimulating male sexual performance (often marketed as "herbal Viagra"), and enhancing athletic performance (as an alternative to anabolic steroids). More recently, however, yohimbe and quebracho have also been showing up in dietary supplements focused toward promoting fat loss and muscle gain at the same time.

A purified extract from yohimbe bark yields yohimbine, which is similar in chemical structure to caffeine and ephedra; it is regulated as a prescription medication for treating erectile dysfunction in males. Yohimbine functions as a monoamine oxidase (MAO) inhibitor to increase levels of the neurotransmitter norepinephrine, but it also acts as a stimulator of the central nervous system, where it interacts with specific receptors (alpha-2 adrenergic receptors) and may increase energy levels and promote fat oxidation.

Although yohimbe is frequently promoted as a natural way to increase testosterone levels for muscle building, strength enhancement, and fat loss, there is no solid scientific proof that yohimbe is either anabolic or thermogenic. Results from a few small trials show that purified synthetic yohimbine can increase blood flow to the genitals, an effect that may occur in both men and women. As such, yohimbe bark, which contains small amounts of natural yohimbine, may be effective in alleviating some mild forms of both "psychological" and "physical" impotence. However, in the few studies conducted on the purified form of yohimbine, only about 30 percent of subjects reported beneficial effects in terms of erectile function and sexual performance.

As the number of yohimbe products on the retail market increases, concerns about their safety are raised because of the reported toxicity of yohimbine. Reported side effects from yohimbe use include minor complaints such as headaches, anxiety, and tension, as well as more serious adverse events, including high blood pressure, heart palpitations, hallucinations, and elevated heart rate. People with high blood pressure and kidney disease should avoid supplements containing yohimbe, and so should women who are, or who could become, pregnant (due to a potential risk of miscarriage). Also, caution should be used when taking yohimbe in combination with certain foods containing tyramine (such as red wine, liver, and cheese) as well as with nasal decongestants or diet aids containing ephedrine or phenylpropanolamine, which could lead to dangerous blood-pressure fluctuations.

Coleus

Coleus (*Coleus forskohlii*) is part of the mint family of plants and has long been used in India, Thailand, and parts of Southeast Asia as both a spice and an Ayurvedic medicine for treating heart ailments and stomach cramps. The roots of the plant are a natural source of forskolin, a compound that can increase cellular levels of cyclic adenosine monophosphate (cAMP), an effect that is theorized to influence many aspects of metabolism. The primary use of coleus extracts in modern dietary supplements is for a purported effect in promoting weight loss and stimulating muscle growth.

The theory behind *Coleus forskohlii* as a dietary supplement is that its content of forskolin can be used to stimulate adenylate cyclase activity, which will increase cAMP levels in the fat cell, in turn activating another enzyme (hormone-sensitive lipase) to start breaking down fat stores. The problem with this theory is that cAMP regulates the activity of hundreds of enzymes in each cell —and those enzymes can be quite different from cell to cell. For example, we know that in cell cultures (test-tube studies), adding forskolin to fat cells will increase cAMP levels and stimulate lipolysis (breakdown of stored triglycerides into free fatty acids). Add that same forskolin to muscle cells, however, and the primary effect is to stimulate glycogenolysis (breakdown of stored glycogen into free glucose units). Add forskolin to liver cells and you get a stimulation of gluconeogenesis (synthesis of blood glucose from amino acid precursors).

Most of the work conducted on the actions of forskolin has been confined to test tubes. There are no published trials showing that the supplement promotes either weight loss or increased lean body mass or any other health benefit in humans, though health food–industry publications frequently tout a small, poorly conducted trial of six overweight women in whom 500 mg of coleus extract per day for eight weeks caused a loss of body fat and an increase in muscle mass. These data are completely useless to us, as there were no blinding of subjects and no placebo control group, so there is no way to determine whether the weight loss was due to the supplement (which is highly unlikely) or to some other factor, such as a change in diet or exercise patterns (far more likely).

The typical dosage recommendations for coleus extracts are in the range of 100–300 mg per day (10–20 percent forskolin), which appears to be more than enough to induce a significant rise in blood levels of cortisol.

SUMMARY: SUPPLEMENTS TO AVOID

I hope the preceding information helps to put some of the "miracle" weight-loss claims about herbal stimulants into proper perspective. Far from being a stand-alone solution for weight maintenance, these supplements—while they offer the benefits of appetite control, enhanced energy levels, and increased caloric expenditure—absolutely must be used within the proper dosage range (and, even better, should be used in conjunction with at least one cortisol controller). At excessive doses, users risk adverse side effects, long-term elevations in cortisol levels, and the associated metabolic changes that can sabotage weight-loss efforts.

But there is good news. The rest of this chapter profiles some of the supplements that are most effective for controlling stress, balancing cortisol levels, and dealing with many of the associated metabolic changes.

VITAMINS AND MINERALS
FOR STRESS ADAPTATION

It almost goes without saying that taking a general multivitamin and mineral supplement is a good idea for anybody who is under stress, maintains a hectic lifestyle, or needs more energy. Every energy-related reaction that takes place in the body, especially those involved in the stress response, relies in one way or another on vitamins and minerals as cofactors to make the reactions go. For example, B-complex vitamins are needed for metabolism of protein and carbohydrate; chromium is involved in utilizing carbohydrates; magnesium and calcium are needed for proper muscle contraction; zinc and copper are required as enzyme cofactors in nearly three hundred separate reactions; iron is needed to help shuttle oxygen through the blood—the list goes on and on.

It is fairly well accepted in the medical community that sub-clinical or marginal deficiencies of essential micronutrients, especially the B vitamins and magnesium, can lead to psychological and physiological symptoms that are related to stress. One study, published in 2000, looked at the effects of a multivitamin/mineral supplement on overall stress levels. The supplement was a water-soluble formula, composed of vitamins C (1,000 mg), B-1 (15 mg), B-2 (15 mg), B-3 (50 mg), B-6 (10 mg), B-12 (10 mcg), biotin (150 mcg), pantothenic acid (23 mg), calcium (100 mg), and magnesium (100 mg). For a period of thirty days, 150 volunteers, who were prescreened for having high levels of stress, consumed the supplement each morning with water, while another 150 "high-stress" volunteers received a placebo pill. Before and after the thirty-day supplementation period, researchers administered a battery of standardized stress tests. The test results showed a statistically different and clinically important improvement in the overall stress index of the volunteers taking the multivitamin/mineral supplement, but the improvements were not indicated in the placebo group. Another study (also a double-blind, placebo-controlled trial) of eighty healthy male volunteers found that twenty-eight days of treatment with a mineral supplement containing calcium, magnesium, and zinc significantly reduced anxiety and sensations of stress. These studies, and dozens like them, support the rationale behind using a general nutritional supplement as an antistress foundation on which to build a solid cortisol-control regimen.

"Stress-Formula" Multivitamins

In an effort to capitalize on the huge market for "stress-reducing" products, many of the large pharmaceutical and dietary-supplement companies have introduced "stress-formula" multivitamin products. These formulations are based on available scientific evidence suggesting that certain nutrients may be needed at levels higher than the RDAs (recommended daily allowances) for optimal support of adrenal function and control of cortisol levels. For example, vitamin C supplementation at a dose of 1,000 mg per day improves the capacity of the adrenals to adapt to surgical stress by normalizing cortisol and ACTH in patients with lung cancer. Thiamin (vitamin B-1) is effective in reducing the typical increase in postsurgical secretion of cortisol from the adrenal glands. In one study, a combination of vitamins C, B-1, and B-6 was able to bring the pattern of cortisol secretion back into normal ranges following surgery. Pantothenic acid (vitamin B-5) is another required nutrient for proper functioning of the adrenal gland. Consumption of pantothenic acid by humans buffers the rise in cortisol during experimental stress, which suggests a potential benefit of vitamin B-5 in controlling the hypersecretion of cortisol during periods of stress. Overall, it makes little difference whether you decide to get your cortisol-controlling nutrients as part of a general multivitamin/mineral product or from a more targeted "stress-tab" sort of formula; the important thing is that you *do* get them.

Without getting bogged down in too many details, I can outline some of the general ways in which essential nutrients (vitamins and minerals) help to counteract the detrimental health effects of chronic stress. For example, magnesium, a mineral that we most often think about in terms of bone health and heart function, has been shown to reduce cortisol levels following exhaustive exercise in healthy male athletes. Zinc, a mineral that we commonly associate with bone health and immune function, is known to alter adrenal metabolism when levels in the diet are either too high or too low. In one study, 25–50 mg of zinc (about two to three times the RDA) resulted in a significant fall in plasma cortisol levels in healthy volunteers (again, following an extreme exercise stress test that typically raises cortisol levels). Chromium, a mineral that we typically think of in terms of its benefits for blood-sugar control and appetite regulation, has been shown to help reduce serum cortisol in livestock (cattle and sheep) exposed to the stress of cross-country transport. In both groups of animals, those receiving chromium supplements also demonstrated a more robust immune-system function, as evidenced by a smaller number of infections than the animals receiving the placebo.

In addition to the observed effects of isolated nutrients on cortisol levels, there are numerous instances of general dietary alterations bearing a positive impact on reducing elevated cortisol levels. For example, one study of sodium restriction documented a drop in urinary levels of cortisol following one week on a sodium-restricted diet. Upon switching back to the higher-sodium diet, researchers observed a 30 percent increase in the body's production of cortisol within a few days. Dietary changes in protein and carbohydrate intake are also known to influence the body's handling of cortisol. In one study of athletes, consumption of an amino-acid solution (100 mg arginine, 80 mg ornithine, 70 mg leucine, 35 mg isoleucine, and 35 mg valine) resulted in a significant suppression of cortisol levels within sixty minutes. When it comes to carbohydrate consumption, numerous studies have demonstrated the cortisol-lowering benefits of carbohydrates, especially when they are consumed during exercise. In one notable study, after ten days on a high-carbohydrate diet, cortisol concentrations were significantly lower than after ten days on a lower-carbohydrate diet. Supplementing one's diet with a carbohydrate-rich sports drink has also been shown to reduce serum cortisol during endurance exercise (compared to a placebo drink). High-fat diets, in contrast, have been shown in rodent studies to impair the body's ability to restore normal cortisol levels following stress.

So there you have it—cortisol metabolism, and indeed the entire underlying stress response, is influenced to a large degree by a person's intake of vitamins, minerals, and other nutrients. Knowing this to be true, a big step you can take in controlling your own stress response is to eat right and to take at least a basic multivitamin supplement (or even better, a comprehensive multivitamin/multimineral supplement). For more targeted cortisol-control activity, some nutrients appear to offer additional benefits; these are outlined in the sections that follow.

Vitamin C

Vitamin C, also known as ascorbic acid, is a water-soluble vitamin needed by the body for hundreds of vital metabolic reactions. As a dietary supplement, vitamin C is consumed by more people than any other vitamin, mineral, or herbal product. Good food sources of vitamin C include all citrus fruits (oranges, grapefruit, lemons) as well as many other fruits and vegetables, such as strawberries, tomatoes, broccoli, Brussels sprouts, peppers, and cantaloupe.

As a dietary supplement, vitamin C is generally regarded as a potent antioxidant and is typically consumed for the prevention of colds, stimulation of the immune system, promotion of wound healing, and to ward off some of the detrimental effects of stress. Because of the wide variety of reactions in which vitamin C plays a role, many claims are made about its value as a supplement. Perhaps the best-known function of vitamin C is as one of the key nutritional antioxidants, whereby it protects the body from free-radical damage. As a water-soluble vitamin, ascorbic acid performs its antioxidant functions within the aqueous portions of the blood and cells, and it can help restore and augment the antioxidant potential of vitamin E (a fat-soluble antioxidant).

As a preventive against infections such as influenza and other viruses, vitamin C is thought to strengthen cell membranes, thereby preventing entrance of the virus to the interior of the cell. Support of immune-cell function is another key role performed by vitamin C and one that may help fight infections in their early stages. The combined effects of cellular strengthening, collagen synthesis, and antioxidant protection are thought to account for the multifaceted approach by which vitamin C helps to counteract stress and maintain health.

In two separate studies about supplementing with vitamin C (1,000–1,500 mg per day for one week), ultramarathon runners showed a 30 percent lower cortisol level in their blood when compared to runners receiving a placebo. In another study of healthy children undergoing treatment with synthetic corticosteroids, 1 gram (1,000 mg) of vitamin C, consumed three times a day for five days, resulted in significantly lower cortisol levels compared to healthy children given a placebo. In a study of lung-cancer patients, a dose of 2 grams of vitamin C, given daily for one week prior to surgery, was able to bring elevated cortisol levels (resulting from the surgery) back to normal ranges in a significantly shorter period of time compared to patients receiving a placebo.

It has been shown in numerous animal and human studies that even a subclinical deficiency of vitamin C (that is, a deficiency so small is doesn't produce results detectable by the usual clinical tests) will result in an elevation of plasma cortisol levels. In studies of various laboratory and livestock animals, even a marginal vitamin C deficiency produced a significant increase in plasma cortisol levels and an inhibition of immune function, both of which were reversed by adding vitamin C back into the diet. These suboptimal levels of vitamin C, and their resulting elevation in cortisol, may account at least in part for the immune-system suppression and mild depression observed in elderly volunteers. In one study, thirty elderly volunteers (ten women and twenty men) were given 1 gram of vitamin C daily for sixteen weeks. Results showed a significant decrease in serum cortisol in both groups, as well as a significant improvement in various parameters of immune function.

Vitamin C supplements are most often used as a way to prevent or reduce the symptoms associated with the common cold—and well over one hundred studies have been conducted in this area. In several of the largest studies, no effect on common-cold incidence was observed, indicating to many scientists that vitamin C has no preventive effects in normally nourished subjects who experience normal exposure to stress. However, a number of smaller, *targeted* studies, conducted on subjects under *heavy stress,* show that vitamin C decreases the incidence of the common cold by more than 50 percent. In other studies, healthy subjects consuming low levels of vitamin C (below 60 mg per day) experienced about one-third fewer colds following vitamin C supplementation.

In most cases, it appears that although the most important and dramatic preventive effects of vitamin C supplementation are experienced by individuals with low vitamin C intakes, those with an average daily consumption from foods may also benefit from supplemental levels—especially during periods of heightened stress. In support of an elevated vitamin C intake, an expert scientific panel recently recommended increasing the current RDA for vitamin C from 60 mg to at least 100–200 mg per day. This same panel also cautioned that taking more than 1,000 mg of vitamin C daily could have adverse effects and recommended that "whenever possible, vitamin C intake should come from fruits and vegetables"—more support for getting at least your "daily five" servings of fruits and vegetables.

Although the Food and Nutrition Board has recently changed the RDA for vitamin C from 60 mg to 75–90 mg (instead of to 100–200 mg per day, as recommended by the expert panel), it is well established that almost everybody can benefit from ingesting even higher levels. For example, the vitamin C recommendation for cigarette smokers is 100–200 mg per day, because smoking destroys vitamin C in the body. You need not worry about developing the vitamin C deficiency disease, scurvy (as long as you consume at least 10 mg of vitamin C daily), but be sure to increase your intake if you're exposed to stress (physical or psychological) or infection (for example, from a sick friend of family member).

In terms of safety, vitamin C is extremely safe even at relatively high doses, because most of the excess is excreted in the urine. At high doses (over 1,000 mg per day), however, some people experience gastrointestinal side effects, such as stomach cramps, nausea, and diarrhea. In addition, vitamin C intakes above 1,000 mg per day may increase the risk of developing kidney stones in some people.

Although vitamin C is well absorbed, the percentage absorbed from supplements decreases with higher dosages; therefore, optimal absorption is achieved by taking several small doses throughout the day. For example, try 100–250 mg per dose for a total daily intake of 250–1,000 mg. Full blood and tissue saturation is typically achieved with intakes of 250–500 mg per day.

Sharon was a high-achieving college student who experienced an extreme degree of anxiety and stress during exams—particularly during midterm and final-exam periods. Like millions of students around the world, Sharon was far more likely to become sick (usually catching a cold or the flu) during exam periods than at other times of the year. During exam periods, the combination of poor diet (lots of junk food), inadequate sleep (late-night study sessions), and heightened anxiety (about her grades) led to a cortisol-induced suppression of immune-system function—and a dramatic rise in illness rates for Sharon and her classmates.

To guard against the inevitable increase in cortisol levels and suppression of immune function during midterm-exam week, Sharon supplemented her diet with a cortisol-controlling blend of vitamin C (250 mg, taken twice daily) and phytosterols (60 mg of beta-sitosterol, taken twice daily), along with a direct immune-boosting dose of echinacea (125 mg, taken twice daily). Unfortunately, she also kept up her steady pre-exam diet of Mountain Dew, M&M's, and inadequate sleep. Despite this less than optimal foundation of diet and sleep for controlling cortisol levels, the supplement regimen appeared to bring Sharon's immune system through midterms with flying colors: She avoided catching a cold during or after her exams that year.

Calcium

Calcium is the most abundant mineral in the human body, and although 99 percent of your body's calcium is stored in the bones, the remaining 1 percent is found in the blood and within cells, where it performs a vital role in dozens of metabolic processes. Research into the effects of calcium on metabolism has revealed the profound impact of calcium in such areas as reducing the risk of colon cancer, cutting symptoms of PMS in half (pain, bloating, mood swings, and food cravings), and controlling blood pressure. If this weren't enough evidence that calcium supplements might be a good idea, there is also some evidence that calcium can even influence mood and behavior. This possibility comes from studies of rats, in which the animals become agitated when fed a low-calcium diet but are more calm and relaxed when their diets contain adequate calcium levels.

You may have noticed the "Got Milk?" advertising campaign in recent years, produced by the National Dairy Council. The obvious purpose of the ads is to convince you to drink more milk and consume more dairy products in general (not a bad idea for most people). Some of these ads depict potential weight-loss benefits from getting your full daily dose of calcium—and the research to support this position has come from several universities across the country. Scientists at the University of Tennessee have found that low calcium intake is associated with elevated cortisol production *within* fat cells. As I discussed in Chapter 4, if you're trying to lose weight, the last thing you want is to develop high levels of cortisol within your fat cells, because it is precisely this cortisol that serves as a potent "fat-storing" signal, especially to the fat cells in your belly region.

Right now you may be thinking, "I already need calcium for strong bones, so I might as well get some more in my diet, just in case it really *can* help with weight control." To that, I'd say, "Great idea!"—and so would researchers from the University of Colorado, Purdue University, and Creighton University. Research from the University of Colorado has shown that subjects with the highest dietary calcium intake (whether from dairy products or calcium supplements) also had the highest calorie expenditure and fat metabolism. Purdue researchers found that the difference between consuming 1,000 mg/day of calcium versus 500 mg/day was as much as twenty pounds of body fat in two years (higher calcium intake leading to lower body fat levels). If all this weren't enough, one of the world's foremost calcium and bone metabolism experts, Dr. Robert Heaney, at Creighton University, in Nebraska, declared in a nutrition journal editorial that simply increasing calcium intake to 1,000–1,500 mg/day could reduce obesity in the population by 60 to 80 percent!

As a dietary supplement, calcium is about as safe as it gets, with side effects being quite rare and modest in severity (occasional constipation at higher intakes). Because practically nobody consumes enough calcium in their daily diet, and with calcium being so cheap and easily available, this is certainly one of the nutrients for which supplementation is most highly recommended.

Magnesium

Magnesium is a mineral that functions as a coenzyme (the active part of an enzyme system) for nerve and muscle function, regulation of body temperature, energy metabolism, DNA and RNA synthesis, and the formation of bones. The majority of the body's magnesium (60 percent) is found in the bones; therefore, many of us tend to think of magnesium as a bone-specific nutrient.

Because magnesium serves as a cofactor for so many regulatory enzymes, particularly those involved with energy metabolism and nervous-system function, magnesium needs may increase during periods of heightened stress. Magnesium is required for proper enzyme function in converting carbohydrates, protein, and fat into energy—and at least a few studies have suggested a potential role for magnesium supplements in energy metabolism by showing increased exercise efficiency in endurance athletes. Although there is no overwhelming evidence to suggest any increases in muscular strength or elevated energy levels following magnesium supplementation, clinical studies have shown that magnesium supplements help lessen feelings of anxiety and overall stress.

The Daily Value (DV, another term for RDA) for magnesium is 400 mg per day, but requirements may be elevated somewhat by stressors such as exercise. Additionally, because magnesium increases calcium absorption, it is recommended that calcium supplements taken for bone building or prevention of bone loss contain magnesium. Food sources of magnesium include artichokes, nuts, beans, whole grains, and shellfish, but since nearly three-quarters of the American population fails to consume enough magnesium, supplements may be warranted—especially during periods of heightened stress. Excessive magnesium intake can cause diarrhea and general gastrointestinal distress, as well as interfere with calcium absorption and bone metabolism (even though optimal levels of magnesium *assist* calcium absorption). Therefore, since no known benefits are associated with consuming more than 600 mg per day of magnesium, higher intakes should be avoided.

Thiamin

Thiamin, also known as vitamin B-1, is a water-soluble vitamin that functions in carbohydrate metabolism to help convert pyruvate to acetyl CoA for entry into the Krebs cycle and subsequent steps to generate ATP. All this is technical talk for saying that thiamin helps give you energy. Thiamin also functions in maintaining the health of the nervous system and heart muscle. Food sources of thiamin include nuts, liver, brewer's yeast, and pork.

Because of thiamin's role in carbohydrate metabolism and nerve function, supplements have been promoted for increasing energy levels and maintaining memory. Thiamin also seems to be involved in the release of the neurotransmitter acetylcholine from nerve cells, and thiamin deficiency is associated with generalized muscle weakness and mental confusion.

Dietary thiamin requirements are based on caloric intake, so individuals who consume more calories, such as athletes, are likely to require a higher than average intake of thiamin to help process the extra carbohydrates into energy. During acute periods of stress, thiamin needs may be temporarily elevated, but outright thiamin deficiencies are rare except in individuals consuming a severely restricted diet.

No adverse side effects are known with thiamin intakes at RDA levels or even at levels several times the RDA, which is 1.5 mg. Virtually every multivitamin contains thiamin at 100 percent RDA levels or higher, with supplements focused on alleviating stress containing two to ten times RDA levels, dosages that are still quite safe.

Riboflavin

Riboflavin, also known as vitamin B-2, is a water-soluble vitamin that serves primarily as a coenzyme for many metabolic processes in the body, such as the formation of red blood cells and the function of the nervous system. Riboflavin is involved in energy production as part of the electron transport chain that produces cellular energy. As a building block for FAD (flavin adenine dinucleotide), riboflavin is a crucial component in converting food into energy. FAD is required for electron transport and ATP production in the Krebs cycle. Liver, dairy products, dark-green vegetables, and many seafoods are good sources of riboflavin.

Requirements for riboflavin, like most B vitamins, are related to calorie intake—so the more food you eat, the more riboflavin you need to support the metabolic processes that will convert the food into usable energy (but by eating the right foods, such as dairy products and veggies, you'll also be getting more riboflavin). Women should be aware that riboflavin needs are elevated during pregnancy and lactation, as well as when taking oral contraceptives (birth-control pills). Athletes may require more riboflavin due to both increased caloric intake and increased energy needs induced by exercise, which the body perceives as a stressor.

There is no strong support for the efficacy of isolated riboflavin supplements in promoting health outside of correcting a nutrient deficiency. Despite the role of riboflavin in a variety of energy-generating processes, the chances of a supplement improving energy levels in a well-nourished person is unlikely, but those individuals under high levels of emotional or physical stress may have increased requirements.

No serious side effects have been reported for supplementation with riboflavin at levels several times above the DV of 1.7 mg. Because the body excretes excess riboflavin in the urine, high supplemental levels are likely to result in fluorescent-yellow urine.

Pantothenic Acid

Pantothenic acid, also known as vitamin B-5, is a water-soluble vitamin widely distributed in most animal and plant foods. It is physiologically active as part of two coenzymes: acetyl coenzyme A (CoA) and acyl carrier protein. Pantothenic acid functions in the oxidation of fatty acids and carbohydrates for energy production, as well as in the synthesis of fatty acids, ketones, cholesterol, phospholipids, steroid hormones, and amino acids. Food sources of pantothenic acid include liver, egg yolk, fresh vegetables, legumes, yeast, and whole grains. Because it is found in many foods, a deficiency is extremely rare in people who consume a varied diet.

Vitamin B-5 is often referred to as an "antistress" vitamin because of its central role in adrenal-cortex function and cellular metabolism. Unfortunately, there is limited evidence from controlled studies to suggest that pantothenic acid taken on its own will reduce feelings of stress and anxiety or provide protection during times of stress. Therefore, it probably makes more sense to consume vitamin B-5, along with the other B-complex vitamins, as part of a balanced blend of all the essential nutrients, because there *is* good cortisol-control data for mixtures of B vitamins that include B-5.

As a water-soluble B vitamin, B-5 is generally considered a safe supplement, but large doses (10 grams or more) may cause diarrhea. Additional supplementation beyond the levels found in a multivitamin blend (5–50 mg per day) is probably unnecessary.

Pyridoxine

Pyridoxine, also known as vitamin B-6, is a water-soluble vitamin that performs as a cofactor for about seventy different enzyme systems, most of which have something to do with amino acid and protein metabolism. Because vitamin B-6 is also involved in the synthesis of neurotransmitters in the brain and nerve cells, it is frequently recommended as a nutrient to support mental function (mood) and nerve conduction, especially during periods of heightened stress. Some athletic supplements include vitamin B-6 because of its role in the conversion of glycogen to glucose for energy in muscle tissue. Food sources of pyridoxine include poultry, fish, whole grains, and bananas.

Because vitamin B-6, like most of the B vitamins, is involved as a cofactor in such a wide variety of enzyme systems, claims can be made for virtually any health condition. For example, because B-6 is needed for the conversion of the amino acid tryptophan into niacin, a common B-6 claim relates to healthy cholesterol levels, because niacin can help lower cholesterol in some people. Because B-6 also plays a role in prostaglandin synthesis, claims are often made for B-6 in regulating blood pressure, heart function, and pain levels, each of which is partially regulated by prostaglandins. Vitamin B-6 needs are increased in individuals consuming a high-protein diet, as well as in women taking oral contraceptives (birth-control pills).

Vitamin B-6 supplements, in conjunction with folic acid, have been shown to have a significant effect in reducing plasma levels of homocysteine (an amino acid metabolite linked to increased risk of atherosclerosis). In many animal models of hypertension, supplemental pyridoxine lowers blood pressure, and there is preliminary evidence for antihypertensive activity in humans as well. Additionally, we know that physiological levels of pyridoxal phosphate (PLP, the active form of B-6) interact with glucocorticoid (cortisol) receptors to down-regulate their activity—suggesting that B-6 supplements may be able to favorably counteract some of the adverse effects of elevated cortisol levels.

Numerous animal studies have shown that animals subjected to various stressors have an increased incidence of gastric ulcers. Animals supplemented with pyridoxine tend to have fewer stress-induced ulcers compared to animals given placebo. In one notable study of rabbits exposed to hypoxic stress (resulting from high altitude and reduced oxygen levels), pyridoxine feeding was shown to reduce plasma levels of cortisol by as much as 55 percent.

As a water-soluble B vitamin, pyridoxine is generally very safe as a dietary supplement. Excessive intakes (2–6 grams acutely or 500 mg chronically) are associated with sensory neuropathy (loss of feeling in the extremities), which may or may not be reversible. The RDA for vitamin B-6 is only 2 mg per day, an amount contained in virtually all multivitamin supplements. Pregnant and lactating women should not take more than 100 mg of vitamin B-6 per day.

SUMMARY: VITAMINS AND MINERALS

When it comes to dietary supplementation for stress adaptation and cortisol control, the first line of defense appears in the form of a comprehensive multivitamin/multimineral supplement (MVMS). The most effective choices will be those products that offer a balanced blend of the key vitamins and minerals the body needs during the stress response. In particular, vitamin C, magnesium, and the full B-complex group are probably most important from the standpoint of their direct involvement in the body's stress response, but all of the essential and semiessential vitamins and trace minerals are needed as well. A comprehensive MVMS, when used as part of a regimen of balanced diet and regular exercise, represents the antistress foundation on which you can add the targeted cortisol-control supplements that are covered in sections to come.

CORTISOL-CONTROL SUPPLEMENTS

The preceding section outlined the importance for everybody of establishing a sound antistress foundation through the use of a balanced multivitamin supplement. For some people, this general nutritional foundation will be enough to help maintain a normal cortisol profile and stress response. For most others, however, a more targeted cortisol-controlling supplementation regimen may be needed to directly modulate the stress response and control cortisol levels within a healthy range.

For example, the "Stressed Jesses" among us will certainly need a *daily* cortisol-control regimen—and they'll need to follow it very closely. "Strained Janes" will also benefit from their own cortisol-control regimen, but they have the luxury of being somewhat less strict, so missing a day of cortisol control is not the end of the world. "Relaxed Jack" might only need to think about controlling his cortisol levels on an infrequent basis, such as during the rare times when he is under heightened stress. This section outlines some of the most promising supplements for directly modulating the stress response and helping to bring cortisol levels into a more healthful range.

Magnolia Bark

Magnolia bark (*Magnolia officinalis*) is a traditional Chinese medicine used since A.D. 100 for treating stagnation of *qi* (low energy) as well as a variety of syndromes, such as digestive disturbances caused by emotional distress and emotional turmoil. (In China it is known as *houpu* or *hou po*.) Magnolia bark is rich in two biphenol compounds, magnolol and honokiol, which are thought to contribute to the primary antistress and cortisol-lowering effects of the plant. The magnolol content of magnolia bark is generally in the range of 2–10 percent, while honokiol tends to occur naturally at 1–5 percent in dried magnolia bark. Magnolia bark also contains a bit less than 1 percent of an essential oil known as *eudesmol,* which is classified as a triterpene compound, and may provide some additional benefits as an antioxidant.

Two of the most popular herbal medicines used in Japan, one called *saiboku-to* and another called *hange-kobuku-to,* contain magnolia bark and have been used for treating ailments from bronchial asthma to depression to anxiety. Japanese researchers have determined that the magnolol and honokiol components of *Magnolia officinalis* are one thousand times more potent than alpha-tocopherol (vitamin E) in their antioxidant activity, thereby offering a potential heart-health benefit. Other research groups have shown both magnolol and honokiol to possess powerful "brain-health" benefits via their actions in modulating the activity of various neurotransmitters and related enzymes in the brain (increased choline acetyltransferase activity, inhibition of acetylcholinesterase, and increased acetylcholine release).

Numerous animal studies have demonstrated that honokiol acts as a central-nervous-system depressant at high doses, but as an anxiolytic (antianxiety and antistress) agent at lower doses. This means that a small dose of honokiol, or a magnolia bark extract standardized for honokiol content, can help to de-stress a person, while a larger dose might have the effect of knocking her out.

When compared to pharmaceutical agents such as Valium (diaze-pam), honokiol appears to be as effective in its antianxiety activity, yet not nearly as powerful in its sedative ability. These results have been demonstrated in at least half a dozen animal studies and sug-gest that magnolia-bark extracts standardized for honokiol content would be an appropriate approach for controlling the detrimental effects of everyday stressors without the tranquilizing side effects of pharmaceutical agents.

No significant toxicity or adverse effects have been associated with the traditional use of magnolia bark, which is as a decoction (hot-water tea) using 3–9 grams of dried bark (and only obtained via a practitioner of traditional Chinese medicine). Extracts of magnolia bark are now available in commercial antianxiety prod-ucts; these come in a powdered or pill form at doses of 250–750 mg per day and standardized to 1–2 percent honokiol and magnolol.

Researchers in California and Florida studying "stress-eaters" have recently shown that while magnolia bark extract can reduce some indicators of stress and anxiety, there is no significant effect on either daytime cortisol levels or body weight. However, mag-nolia does appear to have a small effect on reducing *evening* corti-sol levels—which suggests a potential benefit on enhancing sleep quality.

> *Rachel,* the single mom in Chapter 6 who suffered from stress-related irritability and anxiety, was an avid fitness walker and vegetarian. As such, she already had the diet and exercise part of her cortisol-control regimen well covered. By adding a twice-daily supplement of magnolia bark extract (150 mg in the A.M. and 300 mg in the P.M.), she was able to reduce a great deal of her perceived stress, anxiety, and irritability. Rachel reported feeling more "balanced" and relaxed.

Theanine

Theanine is an amino acid found in the leaves of green tea (*Ca-mellia sinensis*). Theanine offers quite different benefits from those imparted by the polyphenol and catechin antioxidants for which green tea is typically consumed. In fact, through the natural production of polyphenols, the tea plant converts theanine into catechins. This means tea leaves harvested during one part of the growing season may be high in catechins (good for antioxidant benefits), while leaves harvested during another time of year may be higher in theanine (good for antistress and cortisol-controlling effects). Theanine is unique in that it acts as a nonsedating relaxant to help increase the brain's production of alpha waves. This makes theanine extremely effective for combating tension, stress, and anxiety—without inducing drowsiness. Clinical studies show that theanine is effective in dosages ranging from 50 to 200 mg per day. Three to four cups of green tea are expected to contain 100–200 mg of theanine.

In addition to being considered a relaxing substance (in adults), theanine has also been shown to provide benefits for improving learning performance (in mice), and promoting concentration (in students). No adverse side effects are associated with theanine consumption, making it one of the leading natural choices for promoting relaxation without the sedating effects of depressant drugs and herbs. When considering the potential benefits of theanine as an antistress or anticortisol supplement, it is important to distinguish its nonsedating relaxation benefits from the tranquilizing effects of other relaxing supplements such as valerian and kava, which are actually mild central-nervous-system depressants.

As mentioned above, one of the most distinctive aspects of theanine activity is its ability to increase the brain's output of alpha waves. Alpha waves are one of the four basic brain-wave patterns (delta, theta, alpha, and beta) that can be monitored using an electroencephalogram (EEG). Each wave pattern is associated with a particular oscillating electrical voltage in the brain, and the different brain-wave patterns are associated with different mental states and states of consciousness (see Table 8.1 on the next page).

Alpha waves, which indicate what we call "relaxed alertness," are nonexistent during deep sleep as well as during states of very high arousal such as fear or anger. During deep sleep, the predominant brain waves are the slow delta waves (0–4 cycles/second). When we are in light sleep, or merely drowsy, the slightly faster theta waves are the most prevalent (4–8 cycles/second). Beta waves, which have the fastest cycle rates at 13–40 cycles/second, appear during highly stressful situations, when most of us find it difficult to concentrate or focus on anything. Alpha waves, at 8–13 cycles/second, are slower than high-stress beta waves, but faster than the delta and theta waves associated with sleep. They are the predominant brain-wave pattern seen during wakefulness, when a person is engaged in relaxed and effortless alertness. In other words, alpha waves are associated with your highest levels of physical and mental performance; therefore, you want to maximize the amount of time during your waking hours that your brain spends in an alpha state.

Table 8.1: Brain-Wave Oscillation Patterns

Brain-Wave Pattern	Cycles per Second	Mood/State of Consciousness
Delta	0–4	Deep sleep (stages 3 and 4)
Theta	4–8	Drowsy/light sleep (stages 1 and 2)
Alpha	8–13	Relaxed/wakeful/alert
Beta	13–40	Stressed/anxious/difficulty concentrating

An interesting analogy for emphasizing the importance of the different types of brain waves is to compare them to the gears of a car: The slowest brain waves (delta and theta) represent the "idling" and "getting started" gears, alpha acts as the primary "working gear," and beta functions as the fastest "hyperdrive" gear, where you might be spinning your wheels instead of getting anywhere. Just as you use different gears in your car for different driving conditions, your brain generates different wave patterns when it is engaged in different activities. For example, too few theta and delta waves means that you're likely to suffer from insomnia, while too many would cause you to stumble around in a constant drowsy fog. The best situation is to experience an orderly process from one brain-wave pattern to the next—from restful sleep (delta/theta) to focused alertness (alpha) and back to restful sleep (theta/delta)—throughout a twenty-four-hour period. You'll notice that beta has been left out of the ideal cycle, because we don't need to experience anger or agitation if we can avoid it.

Unfortunately, our high-stress modern lifestyles result in the majority of us skipping our second and third brain gears (theta and alpha). Many people wake up suddenly out of a deep sleep (delta) at the sound of an alarm clock, which induces immediate stress and anxiety (beta) about being late or being under time pressure. After insufficient sleep, we use stimulants (caffeine) to force us into an artificial wakefulness that promotes beta waves (and higher cortisol levels) while suppressing both theta and alpha waves (and inhibiting cortisol reduction). For much of the day, the combined effects of work stress and time urgency have us swimming in beta waves and high cortisol levels. By the time we finally get to bed at night, we're so exhausted that we completely bypass the unwinding benefits of theta sleep (when cortisol levels fall) and instead fall unconscious into the deeper (delta) stages of sleep, but rarely for long enough.

Why is all this talk about brain waves important? Because this constant charging back and forth between delta and beta waves tends to keep cortisol levels elevated throughout the daylight hours (a bad thing) while also disallowing time for those levels to subside during the night (a *really* bad thing). In terms of our mental and physical performance, a constant lack of theta and alpha waves means that we can't concentrate (alpha) when we need to, and we can't relax (theta) when we want to.

And this is where theanine comes in. By increasing the brain's output of alpha waves, theanine can help us to "rebalance" our brain-wave patterns, as well as help to control anxiety, increase focus and concentration, promote creativity, and improve overall mental and physical performance. Research studies are quite clear about the facts that people who produce more alpha brain waves also have less anxiety, that highly creative people generate more alpha waves when faced with a problem to solve, and that elite athletes tend to produce a burst of alpha waves on the left side of their brain during their best performances.

Pretty good stuff—and the best way to increase your output of alpha waves is via theanine consumption. This can easily be accomplished by consuming three to four cups of green tea each day (theanine counteracts a fair portion of the adverse stimulant effect of caffeine), or by taking a daily theanine supplement (50–200 mg per day). Before you decide to use decaffeinated green tea as a source of theanine, be aware that most of the theanine is lost during the decaffeination process, so if you wish to avoid caffeine entirely, a supplement may be your most reliable source. Theanine supplements are available in capsule or tablet form as pure (synthetic) theanine, and as a natural extract from green tea (enriched to as much as 20–35 percent theanine). Because theanine reaches its maximum levels in the blood between thirty minutes and two hours after taking it, it can be used both as a daily cortisol-control regimen and "as needed" during stressful events.

Epimedium

The use of epimedium as a medicinal herb dates back to at least A.D. 400. It has been used as a tonic for the reproductive system (boosting libido and treating impotence) and as a rejuvenating tonic (to relieve fatigue). Animal studies have shown that epimedium may function a bit like an adaptogen (more on adaptogens appears later in the chapter) by increasing levels of epinephrine, norepinephrine, serotonin, and dopamine when they are low (an energy-promoting effect), and by reducing cortisol levels when they are elevated (an antistress effect). There is also evidence that epimedium can restore low levels of both testosterone and thyroid hormone to their normal levels; this may account for some of the benefits of epimedium in improving libido (sex drive). Animal studies using epimedium have shown a reduction in bone breakdown, an increase in muscle mass, and a loss of body fat—each of which may be linked to the observed reduction of elevated cortisol to normal levels.

In a series of studies conducted in humans and animals by Chinese researchers, immune-system function was directly suppressed and bone loss was accelerated by using high-dose synthetic cortisol (glucocorticoid drugs). Subsequent administration of epimedium extract reduced blood levels of cortisol and improved immune-system function (in the humans) and slowed bone loss and strengthened bones (in the animals).

It is interesting to note that although at least fifteen active compounds have been identified in epimedium extracts (luteolin, icariin, quercetin, and various epimedins), many supplement companies currently use extracts standardized only for icariin. The traditional use of epimedium is as a hot-water decoction (tea), which would result in a very different profile of active constituents when compared to the high-icariin alcohol extracts that are more commonly used in commercial products. Although at least one testtube study has shown icariin to protect liver cells from damage by various toxic compounds, other feeding studies (in rodents) have suggested that high-dose icariin may be associated with kidney and liver toxicity.

Because all of the existing scientific evidence for the antistress and cortisol-controlling effect of epimedium has been demonstrated for water-extracted epimedium (that is, as a tea), and because this form of extraction may result in a safer form of epimedium (compared to the high-icariin alcohol extract), it may be prudent to select supplements that specifically use a more traditional formulation. Commercial preparations of the water-extracted form of epimedium will indicate on their labels that they are water-extracted, while the more concentrated (high-icariin) alcohol extracts tend to emphasize their icariin content (usually 20 percent or so). There have been no reports of adverse side effects associated with the traditional, water-extracted preparation of epimedium at the suggested dosage (250–1,000 mg per day for cortisol control).

You may remember *Holly* and *Alan* as the young newlyweds mentioned in Chapter 6 whose high-achievement, high-stress lives resulted in a disconcerting loss of libido. Both exercised religiously (four to five times each week), but their diets needed some tweaking; specifically, each needed a better balance of carbs with proteins, more fresh fruits and veggies, and to adopt more regular eating patterns. Along with these nutritional recommendations, they both started on a supplement regimen of epimedium (300 mg per day) and DHEA (25 mg per day for Holly and 50 mg per day for Alan).

After about one week on the supplements, Holly and Alan were grinning from ear to ear (we need not go into the details why). The combination of epimedium and DHEA helped to normalize their cortisol-to-DHEA ratios as well as their libidos, putting the spark back into their sex life.

Phytosterols

Phytosterols include hundreds of plant-derived sterol compounds (including sterols and sterolins) that bear structural similarity to the cholesterol made in our bodies, but none of the artery-clogging effects. The most prevalent phytosterols in the diet are beta-sitosterol (BS), campesterol, and stigmasterol. Plant oils contain the highest concentration of phytosterols, so nuts and seeds have fairly high levels, and all fruits and vegetables generally contain some. Perhaps the best way to obtain phytosterols is to eat a diet rich in fruits, vegetables, nuts, and seeds—which obviously would bring numerous other benefits as well.

Phytosterols appear to help modulate immune function, inflammation, and pain levels through their effects on controlling the production of inflammatory cytokines. This modulation of cytokine production and activity may also help to control allergies and reduce prostate enlargement. In athletes competing in marathons and other stressful endurance events, phytosterols are known to reduce cortisol levels, maintain DHEA levels, and prevent the typical suppression of immune-system function seen after such events. From test-tube and animal studies, it appears that phytosterols such as beta-sitosterol can influence the structure and function of cell membranes in both healthy and cancerous tissue. This effect is known to alter cellular signaling pathways that regulate tumor growth and apoptosis (cell death); it provides a possible explanation for the stimulation of immune function observed following beta-sitosterol supplementation.

In several animal studies examining the effect of beta-sitosterol consumption on experimentally induced breast cancer, the animals fed phytosterols (including beta-sitosterol) showed a dramatic reduction in tumor size (30–80 percent) and a 10–30 percent lower incidence of metastases to the lymph nodes and lungs compared to a control group. From these animal studies, there is strong preliminary evidence that dietary phytosterols do indeed retard the growth and spread of breast cancer cells.

In terms of general immune function, beta-sitosterol has been shown in humans to normalize the function of T-helper lymphocytes and natural killer cells following stressful events, such as marathon running, that normally suppress immune-system function. In addition to alleviating much of the postexercise immune suppression that occurs following endurance competitions, beta-sitosterol has also been shown to normalize the ratio of catabolic stress hormones (i.e., those that break down tissue, such as cortisol) to anabolic (rebuilding) hormones such as DHEA.

In one small study, seventeen endurance runners completed a sixty-eight-kilometer run (about forty miles) and afterward received either 60 mg of beta-sitosterol (nine runners) or a placebo (eight runners) for four weeks. Those runners receiving the beta-sitosterol supplements showed a significant drop in their cortisol-to-DHEA ratio (indicating less stress) as well as reduced inflammation and a markedly lower immunosuppression. Using the ultramarathon as a model for overall stress, researchers concluded that beta-sitosterol is effective in modulating the stress response by managing cortisol levels within a more normal range.

Phytosterols are generally regarded as quite safe because of their widespread distribution in fruits and vegetables. No significant side effects or drug interactions have been reported in any of the studies investigating beta-sitosterol. The typical dosage recommended to achieve the best cortisol-control and immune-function benefits is 100–300 mg per day of a mixed phytosterol blend, including 60–120 mg per day of beta-sitosterol. A handful of roasted peanuts or a couple of tablespoons of peanut butter contain about 10–30 mg of beta-sitosterol, so a few handfuls of Planter's nuts or a scoop of Skippy will supply an effective dose of immune enhancement following exercise (but also a whopping dose of calories).

Because phytosterols afford other health benefits in addition to their role in cortisol control, they are often found in commercial supplements designed for lowering cholesterol, boosting immune function, and maintaining prostate health. Almost always, the phytosterols will be combined with additional ingredients to enhance the primary effect (for example, they might be blended with echinacea in immune-boosting products).

Phosphatidylserine

Phosphatidylserine (PS) is a phospholipid—meaning that it is composed of fatty acids (lipids) and phosphate. PS is concentrated in the brain cells, where it is thought to be related to brain-cell function, but it is also found in *all* cell membranes, where it is thought to play key roles in muscle metabolism and immune-system function. PS has also been shown to modulate many aspects of cortisol overproduction, especially following intense exercise.

There is ample scientific evidence that PS supplementation, in a dose of 100–300 mg per day, can help improve mental function and decrease feelings of depression, even in cases as severe as Alzheimer's disease and other forms of age-related mental decline. More recent studies from Italy have shown much larger doses of PS (400–800 mg per day) to reduce cortisol levels by 15–30 percent following heavy exercise. Because cortisol is catabolic toward muscle tissue (that is, it leads to protein breakdown and muscle loss), athletes frequently use PS supplements to help promote recovery from exercise and decrease slow muscle loss. And because of its benefits in improving cognitive function, PS could also be considered a general antistress nutrient, providing benefits not only for athletes subjected to the physical stress of exercise, but also for individuals who are under chronic emotional stress from hectic lifestyles, job deadlines, and many of the other stresses of a modern, Type C lifestyle.

There do not appear to be any significant side effects associated with dietary supplements containing phosphatidylserine, but due to concerns about mad-cow disease, it is generally recommended to select PS supplements derived from soybeans versus those extracted from cows' brains.

Concentrated PS supplements are available in doses of 50–100 mg per day, and they are quite expensive. For brain and mental support, 100–500 mg per day of PS is recommended for a month or so, followed by a lower maintenance dose of approximately 50–100 mg per day. Athletes may need as much as 800 mg per day immediately before or after intense training to help suppress cortisol secretion and promote muscle recovery. This amount of PS would cost several hundred dollars per month, making these levels less than viable for the average consumer.

Ken was an avid runner, regularly competing in 10K races and occasional marathons. Frustrated with his apparent inability to fully recover between strenuous workouts and intense competitions, despite a regimen of active rest and balanced nutrition, Ken turned to a combination of supplements that included phosphatidylserine (PS) and beta-sitosterol (BS). Both PS and BS have been shown to help athletes reduce the rise in cortisol that is seen during intense exercise. Because elevated cortisol levels are catabolic toward connective tissues such as muscle, tendons, and ligaments—that is, they accelerate the breakdown of these tissues—keeping cortisol levels from rising too high during exercise can be an effective strategy for reducing tissue breakdown and enhancing the repair process.

The combination of PS (50 mg per day) with BS (200 mg per day), taken immediately following each workout, helped Ken's body to control cortisol levels and accelerate his postexercise recovery. The primary end benefit for Ken was a heightened ability to train intensely without getting injured and, thus, to improve his overall performance in his races.

Tyrosine

Tyrosine is an amino acid that has been studied by the U.S. military as a potential antistress nutrient to help soldiers cope with the stress of battle. Findings from several studies suggest that dietary tyrosine supplements can help to reduce the acute effects of stress and fatigue on physical and mental performance. Chronic stress can reduce brain levels of neurotransmitters such as epinephrine, norepinephrine, and dopamine, a phenomenon thought to be related to some of the decline in mental and physical performance during stressful events. Because the brain uses tyrosine to synthesize these neurotransmitters, dietary supplements of tyrosine can help slow their depletion and reduce the declines in performance that are often noted during stressful events. And because neurotransmitters play a role in overall brain function, including depression and other mood disorders, tyrosine supplementation has been studied for its effects on stress, mental function, and Alzheimer's disease.

In soldiers, this theory has been proven under conditions of combat training, sleep deprivation, cold exposure, and extremes of physical exercise. Studies of military cadets undergoing combat training showed that 2,000 mg of tyrosine aided memory and cognitive ability during stress. In other (nonsoldier) studies, tyrosine supplements (100–200 mg per day) were able to offset declines in performance and ability to concentrate in volunteers exposed to stressful situations such as shift work, sleep deprivation, and fatigue.

In animals, dietary tyrosine supplementation has been shown to improve learning ability and memory (ability to navigate a maze), while tyrosine depletion has led to decreased performance, probably via suppressed norepinephrine levels. Tyrosine and norepinephrine levels are often reduced in people with depression or under conditions of stress, and in some forms of obesity. In animal experiments, tyrosine supplementation leads to a slight elevation in oxygen consumption, suggesting an effect on increasing metabolic rate.

In one human study, 6–8 grams of tyrosine or a placebo was given to volunteers subjected to a cardiovascular stress test. Those receiving the tyrosine supplements showed improvements in attention and cognitive function compared to the placebo group. In another study, subjects were given either a placebo or 6–7 grams of tyrosine, in random order on two consecutive days. One hour later, subjects were asked to perform a number of stress-sensitive tasks while simultaneously being exposed to a stressor (loud noise). During the tyrosine supplementation, subjects showed improved performance and decreased blood pressure throughout the study period. In an additional double-blind, placebo-controlled cross-over study, subjects receiving 6–7 grams of tyrosine showed a significant improvement in stress symptoms, mood disturbances, and performance impairments during exposure to extreme stress (four and a half hours of cold and low oxygen). Overall, these studies suggest that tyrosine is effective in modulating the stress response in a variety of stressful conditions.

Since tyrosine is relatively abundant in foods containing protein, it is unlikely that tyrosine supplementation at the levels commonly available would cause significant side effects. Human studies have been conducted with 6–8 grams of tyrosine per day, with no adverse effects noted. (Because of the high cost of tyrosine supplements, commercially available products tend to provide no more than a few hundred milligrams—that is, less than 10 percent of the levels shown to be effective against stress in clinical studies.) Extremely high doses of any isolated amino acid are not recommended, however, as they may cause unpleasant gastrointestinal side effects such as diarrhea, nausea, and vomiting, as well as headaches and nervousness.

Branched-Chain Amino Acids

The group of amino acids referred to as the *branched-chain amino acids* (BCAAs) is comprised of three essential amino acids: valine, leucine, and isoleucine. The recommended intake for the BCAAs is about 3 grams per day, an amount that should be easily obtained from protein foods. Supplemental levels have been used at doses from 3 grams to more than 20 grams per day to increase endurance, reduce fatigue, improve mental performance, increase energy levels, prevent immune-system suppression, and counteract muscle catabolism following intense exercise.

In numerous studies of athletes, BCAAs have been shown to maintain blood levels of glutamine, an amino acid used as fuel by immune-system cells. During intense exercise, glutamine levels typically fall dramatically, removing the primary fuel source for immune cells and leading to a general suppression of immune-system activity (and an increased risk of infections) following the exercise. By supplementing with either glutamine or BCAAs, a person can maintain blood levels of glutamine and thereby avoid suppression of immune-cell activity due to a lack of fuel.

In related studies, BCAA supplements have been shown to bear a beneficial effect on counteracting the rise in cortisol and the drop in testosterone that is often seen in endurance athletes undergoing stressful training. In these studies, intense exercise is used as a model for high stress, so the increased cortisol levels and the reduced testosterone levels are exactly what happen in the rest of us when we experience a stressful situation at work, at home, or while standing in line at the grocery store.

Supplemental intakes of the BCAAs (3–20 grams per day) have been studied in tablet and liquid form with no reported adverse side effects, aside from minor gastrointestinal complaints. Higher intakes should be avoided due to the possibility of blocking the absorption of other amino acids from the diet and the risk of more severe gastrointestinal distress. Unfortunately, because purified sources of the BCAAs are so expensive, commercial products typically provide only a small fraction of the multigram doses that have been studied for performance and recovery.

SUMMARY: CORTISOL CONTROLLERS

The seven supplements discussed in this section—magnolia bark, theanine, epimedium, phytosterols, phosphatidylserine, tyrosine, and BCAAs—represent the most promising natural compounds for directly controlling stress and modulating cortisol levels. But which of them should you choose? One? Three? All seven? To narrow down your choices, it may be helpful to refer to Table 8.2.

Table 8.2: Dietary Supplements to Directly Control Cortisol Levels: An Overview

Supplement	Benefits	Drawbacks	Overall Rank
Magnolia bark	Cortisol control and general effects as an antianxiety and anti-stress agent	Too much could cause sedation and drowsiness	Primary
Theanine	Modulates brain waves for optimal physical and mental performance during stressful events	None	Primary
Epimedium	Direct cortisol control, especially following the stress of dieting	Alcohol extract may be toxic; choose a water extract	Primary
Phytosterols	Balances cortisol-to-DHEA ratio, especially following exercise stress	None	Primary
Phosphatidylserine (PS)	Direct cortisol-lowering effect, especially after intense exercise	High cost at effective doses	Secondary
Tyrosine	Maintains mental performance and concentration during stressful events	High doses needed	Secondary
Branched-chain amino acids (BCAAs)	Reduce muscle breakdown and immune suppression during exercise stress	High doses needed	Secondary

HSD-BALANCING SUPPLEMENTS

As discussed in Chapter 4, HSD (11 beta-hydroxysteroid dehydro-genase-1) is an enzyme within fat cells that is responsible for converting inactive cortisol into active cortisol, which can then serve as a potent fat-storage signal. As such, you do not want to have an overactive HSD enzyme sabotaging your weight-loss efforts. Remember, too much HSD means too much cortisol *inside* your fat cells and too much fat stored in your belly region.

Every major pharmaceutical company in the world is aggressively developing (and patenting) synthetic products to inhibit the activity of HSD and treat obesity and diabetes—but those drugs are still five to ten years away from reaching the market. Luckily, a number of natural flavonoids are known to inhibit HSD, including those from grapefruit juice (naringenin), licorice (glycyrrhizin), soybeans (daidzein and genistein), apples (quercetin), and Chinese medicinal herbs (magnolia/magnolol, *Perillae frutescens*, *Zizyphus vulgaris*, and *Scutellaria baicalensis*).

A very unique class of flavonoids, known as *polymethoxylated flavones* (PMFs), particularly tangeritin, sinensetin, and nobilitin, represent a class of "super flavonoids," extracted from citrus peels, that exhibit approximately threefold potency compared to other flavonoids. Polymethoxylated flavones are just what they sound like—flavonoid compounds with extra methoxy groups compared to "regular" flavones. Like all flavonoids, the PMFs deliver potent antioxidant and anti-inflammatory activity, but the PMF version is about three times more potent in its ability to reduce both HSD activity and cholesterol levels (clinical studies show a 20–30 percent reduction).

PMFs are wonderfully safe—and at the effective dose of 300 mg daily (see below), users will benefit from the antioxidant and anti-inflammatory effects in addition to the HSD- and cholesterol-reducing effects. Unlike some flavonoids, such as naringin from grapefruit, there are no known risks of drug interactions with citrus-derived PMFs. (Certain grapefruit flavonoids can interfere with the liver enzymes needed to metabolize many prescription drugs.)

Table 8.3: Dietary Supplements for HSD Balance

Supplement	Additional Benefits	Drawbacks	Effectiveness
Naringenin/ naringin (grape-fruit)	Also has antioxidant effects	Can interact with many medications	Low
Glycyrrhizin (licorice)	Also has antiulcer effects	Increases blood pressure	Low
Daidzein/ genistein (soybeans)	Also has postmeno-pausal benefits	None—do not exceed 50mg/day	Moderate
Quercetin (apples, onions)	Also has antioxidant effects	None	Moderate
Magnolol (magnolia bark)	Also has antianxiety effects	Can induce drowsiness at higher doses	High
Perillae frutescens (Chinese basil)	Also has anti-inflamma-tory effects	Can be toxic/hallucinogenic at high doses	Low
Zizyphus vulgaris (jujube berry)	Also has antioxidant effects	None	Low
Scutellaria baicalensis	Also has anti-inflamma-tory effects	None	Moderate
PMFs (citrus peel)	Also has antioxidant and anti-inflammatory effects	None	High

Our lab was the first in the world to use PMFs for inhibiting the activity of HSD, and thus also reducing systemic and local cortisol concentrations (in the liver and adipose tissue), while also promoting blood-sugar control and weight loss. As part of the SENSE Lifestyle Program, we provided supplements of PMFs (with Eurycoma root extract—see below in the section on testosterone) to a group of moderately overweight subjects. The PMFs (300 mg of citrus peel extract/day) reduced cortisol levels by 20 percent, body weight by 5 percent, body fat by 6 percent, and waist circumference by 8 percent over a period of six weeks. A longer twelve-week study showed even better results, with additional beneficial effects on reducing cholesterol (–20 percent), boosting mood (+25 percent), reducing fatigue (–48 percent), and maintaining normal testosterone levels and resting metabolic rate.

TESTOSTERONE-CONTROL SUPPLEMENTS

Why is maintenance of testosterone so important? Because, as explained in Chapter 5, testosterone is cortisol's "alter ego." When cortisol levels go up, testosterone levels go down—and vice versa. This means that keeping testosterone within normal ranges (i.e., keeping it from dropping as would be common with chronic stress such as that arising from trying to lose weight) is an important consideration in maintaining a normal stress response. In addition, testosterone is also important for maintaining mood, mental function, sex drive, muscle mass, and overall metabolic rate.

Aside from helping us look (and feel) lean, fit, and strong (although these are all important), maintaining testosterone levels and muscle mass also means that we maintain energy expenditure (muscle burns the vast majority of calories), reduce risk for osteoporosis (more muscle means denser bones), and protect ourselves from other chronic diseases such as heart disease, diabetes, and syndrome X.

So what supplements are effective for keeping testosterone levels at an optimal level? In answering this question, it is important to distinguish between the *maintenance* of testosterone levels and muscle mass and the *enhancement* of testosterone levels and muscle mass. On the one hand, there are a number of dietary supplements that can *maintain* muscle mass during various periods of high stress, but on the other hand, there are very few (perhaps none) that can *enhance* muscle mass. Only high-dose anabolic steroids can do that effectively.

Numerous scientific and medical reports show quite clearly that high stress (such as extremes of exercise) and elevated cortisol levels lead to a drop in testosterone and a dramatic loss of muscle tissue. High stress causes muscles to break down as a result of a number of factors, including elevated cortisol and suppressed levels of both testosterone and its precursor, DHEA (dehydroepiandrosterone). In cases of high cortisol or low testosterone, or both, we know that reducing cortisol to normal levels and/or increasing testosterone to normal levels produces a dramatic effect on maintaining muscle mass. Importantly, however, it does not appear that reducing cortisol to below-normal levels or increasing testosterone to above-normal levels bears any beneficial effect on enhancing muscle mass (too bad for you bodybuilders out there).

The range of supplements that are commonly touted as *muscle maintainers* or *"anticatabolics"* (because they slow the catabolism, or breakdown, of muscle tissue) provide only a handful of substances that offer any good evidence of effectiveness: DHEA, eurycoma, zinc, cordyceps, conjugated linoleic acid (CLA), and HMB (hydroxymethylbutyrate). These are described below.

DHEA

DHEA (dehydroepiandrosterone) is a hormone produced in the adrenal glands, the same glands that produce cortisol. In the body, DHEA is converted into other hormones such as testosterone, estrogen, progesterone, or cortisol—so too much cortisol often means not enough DHEA or testosterone. DHEA levels are known to decrease with age, particularly after the age of forty, but perhaps as early as ages twenty to thirty; therefore, dietary supplementation with DHEA is typically recommended to slow aging, improve memory, increase sex drive, alleviate depression, boost energy, promote weight loss, and build muscle mass.

DHEA supplementation, at 50–100 mg per day, has been shown to maintain normal testosterone levels (bringing them up from suboptimal levels), increase muscle mass, and improve overall feelings of well-being among a group of forty- to seventy-year-old subjects who took the supplements for six months. Another small study (involving nine elderly men) showed a link between five months of DHEA supplementation (at 50 mg per day) and improvements in markers of immune-system function (lymphocytes, natural killer cells, and immunoglobulins). It is important for us to note, however, that the studies in which DHEA is effective in enhancing muscle mass and immune function have looked at subjects with low DHEA and testosterone levels to begin with; this means the DHEA supplements were restoring them to normal levels. Studies that have looked at healthy young men, with normal DHEA and testosterone levels, have shown no muscle-maintaining or immune-enhancing benefits, and instead they have shown an increase in estrogen levels—a bad thing because of the accompanying risk for increased cancer rates.

In people with low DHEA or low testosterone levels, both of which can result from chronic stress, DHEA supplements appear to be effective at doses ranging from 50 to 100 mg per day. DHEA supplements are one of the most popular muscle-building supplements among fitness enthusiasts. Most often sold in tablet or capsule form, DHEA is also sometimes added to protein powders and other products marketed for improving muscle mass. It is also a common ingredient in commercial products focused on antiaging; its inclusion in these products is intended to counteract the well-known drop in DHEA levels that comes with age. Competitive athletes should be aware of the potential for DHEA supplementation to result in a positive drug test (for steroid use) at International Olympic Committee (IOC) and NCAA-sanctioned events.

Eurycoma

Eurycoma longifolia, a Malaysian root often called "Malaysian ginseng" due to its energy-boosting effects, affords a natural way to bring suboptimal testosterone levels back to within normal ranges. It is also probably the best first-line therapy (before trying synthetic DHEA) for anybody suffering from chronic stress. In traditional Malaysian medicine, eurycoma is used as an antiaging remedy because of its positive effects on energy levels and mental outlook (which are most likely the result of improved testosterone levels).

Eurycoma contains a group of small peptides (short protein chains), referred to as "eurypeptides," that are known to have effects in improving energy status and sex drive. The "testosterone-boosting" effects of eurycoma appear not to have anything to do with stimulating testosterone synthesis, but rather appear to increase the release rate of "free" testosterone from its binding hormone (SHBG, sex hormone–binding globulin). In this way, eurycoma is not so much a testosterone "booster" but rather a "maintainer" of normal testosterone levels (testosterone that your body has already produced and needs to release to become active). This would make eurycoma particularly beneficial for individuals with suboptimal testosterone levels, including those who are dieting for weight loss, middle-aged individuals (because testosterone drops after age thirty), and serious athletes who may be at risk for overtraining.

The vast majority of what we know about eurycoma comes to us from rodent studies, test-tube binding evaluations, and a handful of open-label human feeding trials. In the test-tube binding studies, we find that eurycoma peptides and related compounds do indeed help to release more of the "free" form of testosterone from its binding proteins. In the rodent studies, we have more than a dozen reports of increased energy levels, improved hormonal profiles, and enhanced sex drive. In the limited number of human feeding trials, we see a clear subjective indication of reduced fatigue, heightened energy and mood, as well as a greater sense of well-being in the subjects consuming eurycoma.

Unfortunately, there are very few specific feeding studies conducted on athletes or dieters, two groups that are under severe stress and are perhaps the key customers for eurycoma-based products. There are only two U.S.-based research trials of eurycoma—one on mountain bikers, presented at the International Society of Sports Nutrition, ISSN, Annual Scientific Meeting in 2006; and one on moderately overweight dieters, presented at the North American Association for the Study of Obesity, NASSO, in 2006. These studies used 50–100 mg of eurycoma and found a maintenance of normal testosterone levels in the supplemented dieters (compared to a typical drop in testosterone among nonsupplemented dieters) and the supplemented mountain bikers (compared to a typical drop in nonsupplemented riders).

For a dieter, it would be expected for cortisol (a catabolic hormone) to rise and testosterone (an anabolic hormone) to drop following several weeks of dieting stress. This change in hormone balance (cortisol up and testosterone down) is an important cause of the familiar "plateau" that many dieters reach after six to eight weeks on a weight-loss regimen (when the weight loss stops). By maintaining normal testosterone levels, a dieter could expect to also maintain his or her muscle mass and metabolic rate (versus a drop in both subsequent to lower testosterone levels)—and thus continue to lose weight without hitting the dreaded weight-loss plateau.

For an athlete, the same rise in cortisol and drop in testosterone is an early signal of overtraining—a syndrome characterized by reduced performance, increased injury rates, increased appetite, suppressed immune-system activity, moodiness, and weight gain. Obviously, maintenance of normal testosterone levels could prevent some of these overtraining symptoms as well as help the athlete to recover faster and more effectively from daily training bouts.

There are no reported side effects in animal or human studies of eurycoma. It is important to note that the majority of these studies have been conducted on hot-water extracts of eurycoma (which is the traditional Malaysian preparation). Many of the eurycoma extracts currently on the U.S. market are alcohol extracts, which provide a completely different chemical profile, one that may be less effective and less safe than the studied hot-water extracts.

Typical dosage recommendations, based on traditional use and on the available scientific evidence garnered during studies of dieters and endurance athletes, call for 50–100 mg per day of a water-extracted eurycoma root (standardized to 22 percent eurypeptides).

Zinc

Zinc, which should already be a part of your comprehensive multi-mineral supplement, is an essential trace mineral that functions in the activity of approximately three hundred different enzymes. In terms of testosterone and muscle maintenance, 60 percent of the body's zinc supply is stored in the muscles, and zinc is involved in numerous metabolic reactions related to testosterone production, wound healing, energy production, muscle growth, cellular repair, and reproductive function (especially male fertility). Even a mild zinc deficiency has been linked to reduced testosterone levels, suppressed libido (sex drive), decreased sperm count, depressed immunity, and impaired memory.

Luckily, dietary supplementation with zinc at levels of 15–45 mg per day has been shown to increase testosterone levels back to normal ranges, improve immune function, and restore sex drive. These levels of zinc supplementation should not pose any significant adverse side effects, but zinc supplementation needs to be balanced with copper intake (2 mg of copper for every 15 mg of zinc) to avoid the onset of copper deficiency caused by unbalanced zinc supplementation.

Cordyceps

Cordyceps (*Cordyceps sinensis*) is a Chinese mushroom that has been used for centuries to reduce fatigue, increase stamina, and improve lung function. Traditionally, it was harvested in the spring at elevations above fourteen thousand feet, restricting its availability to the privileged. You may remember news reports of cordyceps from a few years ago when a group of Chinese athletes began suddenly breaking world records in swimming and running events. Many of the athletes had been supplementing their diets with an extract from the cordyceps mushroom (along with turtle-blood soup and anabolic steroids).

Despite the case of the steroid-laced Chinese athletes, several small-scale studies of cordyceps have shown improvements in lung function, suggesting that athletes may benefit from an increased ability to take up and use oxygen. A handful of studies conducted on Chinese subjects have shown increases in libido (sex drive) and restoration of testosterone levels (from low to normal) following cordyceps supplementation. Remember that during stressful events cortisol levels rise while testosterone levels drop. Using cordyceps as a way to normalize these suppressed testosterone levels can help to modulate the cortisol-to-testosterone ratio within a lower (and healthier) range. Many of the claims for cordyceps parallel those of ginseng, because cordyceps is also reported to increase energy levels, sex drive, and endurance performance.

Dietary supplements of cordyceps at levels of 2–4 grams per day are not associated with any significant side effects, although the possibility for a slight blood-thinning effect could reduce blood clotting somewhat. Cordyceps supplements are available primarily in powder and capsule forms at mainstream supplement stores, and the dried mushroom can occasionally be found in herbal pharmacies and from practitioners of traditional Chinese medicine (but it is very expensive in this form).

CLA

Conjugated linoleic acid (CLA) is found primarily in meat and dairy products, but the form of CLA used most commonly in dietary supplements is manufactured from vegetable oils such as sunflower oil. CLA is thought to increase the production of prostaglandins, which are derived from fatty-acid molecules and have been linked to an elevated synthesis of growth hormone and various anticatabolic effects (prevention of muscle breakdown) during periods of high stress. In athletes, increased growth-hormone levels are viewed as beneficial for promoting enhanced muscle growth and strength—but CLA does not appear to *enhance* muscle *growth* as effectively as it may be able to *suppress* muscle *loss* (at least in humans). CLA, via its involvement in prostaglandin metabolism, may also be able to increase blood circulation to the muscles and adipose tissue, an effect that has been suggested to improve muscle function and fat mobilization.

The majority of research on the dietary intake of CLA has been conducted in animals, but newer studies in humans are quite positive. Across the range of studies in rodents and in humans, CLA supplementation has been shown to reduce appetite, lower body weight, and enhance muscle maintenance, especially during active weight loss (viewed by the body as a powerful stressor).

Typical dosage recommendations are 3–6 grams per day. Most people ingest less than 1 gram per day from meat and dairy foods. Because CLA is an oil (liquid), supplements are provided almost exclusively in the form of softgel capsules; taking several large capsules per day is necessary to get an effective dose.

HMB

HMB (hydroxymethylbutyrate) is a metabolite of the amino acid leucine (one of the branched-chain amino acids discussed earlier) that plays a role in regulating protein metabolism. In fact, HMB is thought to be the active form of leucine. HMB is found in the diet in small amounts in some protein-rich foods such as fish and milk. Depending on total protein and leucine intake, HMB production in the body may average about ¼–1 gram per day.

There is some evidence that HMB reduces muscle catabolism and may protect against muscle damage. NASA has evaluated HMB as a dietary approach to preventing the muscle wasting associated with prolonged space flight (talk about a stressful situation!). Exercise studies have shown that 1.5–3 grams of HMB daily during weight training can reduce muscle loss and muscle damage. No side effects have been reported in studies of HMB supplementation, but HMB can be quite expensive to take at these levels, making it less attractive to many people as a general muscle-maintenance supplement. As with DHEA, commercial sources of HMB are typically encapsulated powders marketed to bodybuilders and fitness enthusiasts, but HMB is also frequently added to protein powders and related muscle-building products.

Table 8.4: Dietary Supplements for Testosterone and Muscle-Mass Maintenance

Supplement	Daily Dose	Benefits	Drawbacks	Overall Rank
Eurycoma	50–100 mg	Maintains testosterone levels; boosts energy levels	None	Primary
DHEA	50–100 mg	Maintains testosterone levels	High doses can increase estrogen levels	Secondary
Zinc	15–45 mg	Needed for testosterone synthesis	None; must be balanced with copper	Primary
Cordyceps	1–3 grams	Maintains testosterone levels; improves stamina and endurance	None	Primary
CLA	3–6 grams	Maintains growth-hormone levels	Large doses needed	Secondary
HMB	1.5–3 grams	Reduces muscle break-down	Large doses needed	Secondary

ADAPTOGENS (GENERAL ANTISTRESS SUPPLEMENTS)

One of the primary traditional approaches to dealing with chronic stress involves the use of a class of herbs referred to collectively as *adaptogens.* (An adaptogen is a substance that helps one adapt to stressful situations.) These herbs—most notably ginseng, ashwagandha, schisandra, rhodiola, astragalus, suma, and several Asian mushrooms (reishi, maitake, and shiitake)—are thought to alleviate many symptoms and side effects of chronic stress because they help to bring many metabolic systems back toward normal ranges. While the mechanisms of action for these antistress effects are not completely understood for most adaptogenic herbs (and for suma and the Asian mushrooms there is a lack of Western scientific evidence to support their centuries-old use for treating fatigue, anxiety, and stress), across the studies that *have* been conducted, it is clear that at least part of this adaptogenic response is due to effects of the herbs within the adrenal glands, the same place where cortisol is produced.

A variety of experiments have demonstrated similarities among the various adaptogenic herbs in affecting both the adrenal glands and the HPA axis. (Recall from earlier chapters that the HPA axis is the system of three hormonal glands that together mediate our response to stress.) In animal experiments, the range of compounds isolated from adaptogenic herbs appears to provide a "buffering" or "balancing" action that counteracts an exaggerated adrenal response to stress and reduces cortisol secretion while also stimulating adrenal-gland activity during periods of fatigue and low energy levels.

Ginseng

Ginseng is perhaps the most potent (or at least the best known) of the adaptogens. A strain of ginseng known as *panax ginseng* (also called *Korean ginseng*) provides the most well-substantiated effects. Other forms, such as American and Siberian ginseng, contain some of the same compounds found in the Korean species, but in slightly different proportions that provide slightly different effects in terms of antistress benefits. Numerous animal and human studies show that ginseng can increase energy and endurance, improve mental function (learning and maze tests), and improve overall resistance to various stressors including viruses and bacteria, extreme exercise, and sleep deprivation. Human studies have shown improved immune function and reduced incidence of colds and flu following a month of supplementation with 100 mg per day of panax ginseng. In a handful of studies, ginseng supplementation has also provided benefits in mental functioning in volunteers exposed to stress: improvements in ability to form abstract thoughts, in reaction times, and in scores on tests of memory and concentration. In studies that measure general quality-of-life issues, ginseng supplementation at doses of 100–200 mg per day tends to result in improvements in mood, energy levels, stamina, and overall well-being.

In traditional Chinese medicine (TCM), panax ginseng is used as a tonic herb (a substance used to generally strengthen and invigorate the body) with adaptogenic properties. Some studies of ginseng have shown increased energy levels in fatigued subjects, but the majority of ginseng studies (mostly looking at athletic performance) have shown little to no effect. The differences between study results may be due to the fact that many commercially available ginseng supplements actually contain little or no ginseng at all, because the "real stuff" is very expensive.

Siberian ginseng (*Eleutherococcus senticosus; eleuthero* for short) is not truly ginseng, but it's a close enough cousin to deliver some of the same energetic benefits. Eleuthero is also known as *ciwujia* in popular sports/energy products. The Siberian form of ginseng is generally a less expensive alternative to Asian/Korean or panax ginseng, though it may have more of a stimulatory effect rather than an adaptogenic effect—not necessarily a bad thing if you just need a boost. Often promoted as an athletic performance enhancer, eleuthero may also provide mild to moderate benefits in promoting recovery following intense exercise, perhaps due in part to an enhanced delivery of oxygen to recovering muscles.

The active compounds in ginseng are known as *ginsenosides,* and most of the top-quality ginseng supplements will be standardized for ginsenoside content. It is thought that the ginsenosides interact within the hypothalamic-pituitary-adrenal (HPA) axis to balance the body's secretion of adrenocorticotropic hormone (ACTH) and cortisol. ACTH has the ability to bind directly to brain cells and can affect a variety of stress-related processes in the body.

In general, 100–300 mg per day of properly standardized ginseng can improve general indices of stress and reduce the cortisol-to-testosterone ratio, which is a general gauge of overall stress.

Ginseng is one of the many herbal supplements that can be purchased readily as a whole root, a dried powder, or a standardized extract. Because roots and powders can vary widely in their content of active compounds, the most precise approach to ensure that you are getting an effective product is to use a standardized extract. It is also very important to select your ginseng supplement from a reliable manufacturer, as there are numerous examples of commercial products that provide little or no actual ginseng. Products should be standardized to contain 4–5 percent ginsenosides (for panax ginseng) or 0.5–1.0 percent eleutherosides (for Siberian ginseng). A daily intake of 100–300 mg for three to six weeks is recommended to produce adaptogenic and energetic benefits.

For the most part, plants in the ginseng family are generally considered to be quite safe. There are no known drug interactions, contraindications, common allergic reactions, or toxicity associated with Siberian ginseng, panax ginseng, or American ginseng. However, a word of caution is recommended for individuals with hypertension, as the stimulatory nature of some ginseng preparations has been reported to increase blood pressure. Additionally, individuals prone to hypoglycemia (low blood sugar) should use ginseng with caution due to the reported effects of ginseng to reduce blood-sugar levels.

Ashwagandha

Ashwagandha (*Withania somnifera*) is an herb from India that is sometimes called *Indian ginseng*—not because it is part of the ginseng family, but to suggest energy-promoting and antistress benefits that are similar to the ones attributed to the more well known Asian and Siberian ginsengs. Although very little research has been done on ashwagandha, herbalists and natural-medicine practitioners often recommend the herb to combat stress and fatigue. Traditional use of ashwagandha in Indian (Ayurvedic) medicine is to "balance life forces" during stress and aging.

Commercial ashwagandha products are available in a variety of forms—from tablets and capsules to teas and liquids. Standardized powders provided as tablets or capsules generally provide the most stable and convenient form. General dosage recommendations for ashwagandha range from 500 to 1,000 mg per day of an extract standardized to 1–2 percent withanolides, the herb's primary active component. Withanolides are thought to contribute to the calming effects of ashwagandha during periods of stress and may account for the use of ashwagandha as both a general tonic during stressful situations (where it is both calming and fatigue fighting) and as a treatment for insomnia (where it promotes relaxation).

No long-term safety studies have been conducted on ashwagandha, but no reports of adverse side effects have been reported. Because of the effects of ashwagandha on muscle relaxation and as a mild central nervous system depressant, the herb should not be combined with alcohol or other sedatives, sleep aids, or anxiolytics (antianxiety medications). Pregnant women are advised to avoid ashwagandha due to its reported abortifacient (abortion-inducing) effects and potential to induce premature labor.

> *Tracy* was a nurse in a critical-care hospital unit—and the long hours and irregular sleep schedule were beginning to wear her down. Strangely, despite her extreme level of fatigue when she eventually returned home each night, she had a great deal of trouble relaxing and falling asleep. Tracy tried several over-the-counter sleep remedies without much success, and she hated the hungover feeling they left her with the next morning. By incorporating a daily supplement of ashwagandha (150 mg in the A.M. and 300 mg in the P.M.), Tracy was able to control her feelings of stress while at work, without feeling sleepy, as well as to induce relaxation and restful sleep at night.

Suma

Suma *(Pfaffia paniculata)* is a large ground vine native to Central and South America; it is most notably from Brazil and often called *Brazilian ginseng*. Traditional use of suma has been for improving overall health and as a treatment for virtually every illness, leading to its native name of *para toda* (which literally translates to "for everything"). Modern recommendations for suma include claims of effects as an adaptogen, an immune booster, and a treatment for chronic fatigue and anxiety.

According to most contemporary herbalists, suma is best understood as an adaptogen, a substance that helps one adapt to stress and fight infection. Along with other adaptogens, such as eleuthero, Russian Olympic athletes have used suma in the belief that it will enhance sports performance. In the United States, suma is often recommended as a general strengthener of the body, as well as for treatment of chronic fatigue syndrome, ulcers, anxiety, impotence, and low resistance to illness—each of which is related to stress. Few studies have been conducted on suma, but those that are available (in animals) show an immune-strengthening and sexual-stimulation effect, providing at least a small measure of support for the traditional use of the plant.

The typical dosage of suma is 500–1,000 mg per day during periods of heightened stress, anxiety, or fatigue. Suma is rarely found as a stand-alone commercial product, but is typically combined with other ingredients for targeting a specific condition (e.g., suma might be added to ginger and fiber to treat stress-induced ulcers).

Schisandra

The fruit of the schisandra plant (*Schisandra chinensis*), also known as *wu-wei-wi* and sometimes spelled with a *z* (*schizandra*), has a long history of use in traditional Chinese medicine as an herb capable of promoting general well-being and enhancing vitality. In addition to its traditional uses for promoting energy and alleviating exhaustion and immune-system disturbances caused by stress, schisandra has historically been taken to strengthen the sex organs and promote mental function.

Schisandra is touted as a member of the adaptogen family, along with ginseng and related herbs, because of the presence of compounds thought to balance bodily functions related to stress. Lignans are a main constituent of schisandra and may be responsible for the herb's effects in stimulating the immune system, protecting the liver, increasing the body's ability to cope with stress, and inducing a calming (mild sedative) effect.

A few scientific studies have been conducted to test specific effects resulting from schisandra supplementation. In one study, patients with a certain heart malady (dilated cardiomyopathy) were given a combination of panax ginseng, radix ophiopogonis, and schisandra. The subjects' improvement was measured via an echocardiogram as well as a treadmill tolerance test. After taking the herbal blend for forty days, heart function improved significantly and exercise tolerance increased by more than 67 percent. Studies of exercise have shown schisandra to increase work capacity (in running mice) and lessen the rise in cortisol in athletes undergoing heavy training.

Schisandra is generally considered to be safe and nontoxic when used as directed. Typical dosage recommendations are in the range of 100–500 mg per day. Commercial schisandra supplements may be found as stand-alone products or as blends with multiple ingredients (such as ginseng and rhodiola) targeting energy and performance. Reported side effects resulting from schisandra ingestion include mild indigestion and skin rash. Because schisandra may induce uterine muscle contractions (similar to the effects of ashwagandha), pregnant women should not take the herb.

Rhodiola

Rhodiola (*Rhodiola rosea/Rhodiola crenulata*) comprises several species of plants from the Arctic mountain regions of Siberia. The root of the plant is used medicinally and is also known as *Arctic root* or *golden root* and more recently as *crenulin*. Rhodiola has been used for centuries to treat cold and flulike symptoms, promote longevity, and increase the body's resistance to physical and mental stresses. It is typically considered to be an adaptogen (like ginseng) and is believed to invigorate the body and mind to increase resistance to a multitude of stresses. The key active constituents in rhodiola are believed to be rosavin, rosarin, rosin, and salidroside.

In one open clinical trial, rhodiola rosea extract was effective in reducing or removing symptoms of depression in 65 percent of the patients studied. In another open-label study, twenty-six out of thirty-five men suffering from weak erections or premature ejaculation reported improvements in sexual function following treatment with 100–150 mg of rhodiola rosea extract for three months. In another study, of physicians during nighttime hospital duty, 175 mg per day of rhodiola (standardized to 4.5 mg salidroside) for two weeks resulted in a significant improvement in associative thinking, short-term memory, concentration, and speed of audiovisual perception. An additional study of students undergoing a stressful twenty-day period of exams showed that 50 mg per day of rhodiola alleviated mental fatigue and improved well-being.

Overall, rhodiola rosea extract appears to be valuable as an adaptogen, specifically in increasing the body's ability to deal with a number of psychological and physiological stresses. Of particular value is the theoretical role for rhodiola in increasing the body's ability to take up and utilize oxygen—an effect similar to that of cordyceps (see above)—which may explain some of the nonstimulant "energizing" effects attributed to the plant. Rhodiola is often called the poor-man's cordyceps because of ancient stories in which Chinese commoners used rhodiola for energy because the plants grew wild throughout the countryside, while only the emperor and his immediate family and concubines were allowed access to the rare cordyceps mushroom.

Rhodiola rosea extract is thought to be quite safe. There are no known contraindications or interactions with other drugs or herbs, but potential exists for mild allergic reactions (rashes) in some individuals. General dosage recommendations for rhodiola rosea extract are typically in the range of 300–600 mg per day. Like schisandra, rhodiola can be purchased either as a stand-alone product or in combination with other ingredients.

Astragalus

Astragalus is an herb recommended as much for stimulation of the immune system as for its energy-promoting properties. Perhaps because chronic stress can both deplete energy levels and increase the risk of illness and infection, astragalus may be particularly beneficial in individuals who feel fatigued due to high levels of emotional and physical stress. Athletes in particular may benefit from astragalus supplementation because intense training and competition are often associated with an increased incidence of colds and other upper-respiratory-tract infections, conditions for which astragalus is thought to be most effective.

Astragalus has been used as an herbal tonic for centuries in traditional Chinese medicine (TCM) and in Native American folk medicine. As a tonic, astragalus is used primarily as a "prevention" herb throughout the cold and flu season—a different usage from that associated with the popular herb echinacea, which is best used for early-stage treatment as soon as you feel a cold or the flu coming on. In TCM, astragalus is often combined with other tonic herbs, such as ginseng, cordyceps, or ashwagandha, to keep the immune system humming during periods of high stress.

There have been some clinical tests of astragalus on humans, most of which come from China, wherein the herb appears to stimulate the immune system in patients with infections. At least one clinical trial in the United States has shown astragalus to boost levels of T cells (a type of infection-fighting white blood cell) to near-normal ranges in some cancer patients, suggesting the possibility of a synergistic effect of astragalus with chemotherapy. Most of what we know about astragalus, however, comes from test-tube and animal experiments, which show that it can help fight bacteria and viruses by enhancing various aspects of the body's normal immune response; specifically, it enhances function of specific immune-system cells such as T cells, lymphocytes, and neutrophils. In animal studies, astragalus extracts are effective in preventing infection of mice by the influenza virus, possibly by increasing the phagocytotic activity of the white blood cells of the immune system.

When used as recommended, astragalus has no known side effects, although at high intakes gastrointestinal distress and diarrhea are possible. While astragalus is available as a single-ingredient supplement (250–500 mg per day), it may be even more effective in lower doses (100–200 mg per day) when combined with other immune-stimulating herbs and nutrients.

Table 8.5: Adaptogen Overview

Supplement	Dose (per Day)	Primary Effect
Ginseng (panax and Siberian)	100–300 mg	Increases energy levels
Ashwagandha	500–1,000 mg	Reduces stress perception
Suma	500–1,000 mg	General stress protection
Schisandra	100–500 mg	General antistress effects
Rhodiola	300–600 mg	Increases energy and stamina
Astragalus	250–500 mg	General antistress/immune effects

SUMMARY: ADAPTOGENS

As part of the hierarchy of natural cortisol-controlling compounds, adaptogens certainly represent a powerful and effective solution for counteracting many of the detrimental effects of stress. Within this hierarchy, however, the adaptogenic herbs are probably best thought of as "reinforcements" during periods of particularly high stress.

In this context:

- A solid *foundation* of multivitamin and multimineral supplementation (featuring vitamin C, calcium, magnesium, etc.) is the first step in a good plan for fighting stress.
- The next step should be *targeted* modulation of cortisol, HSD, and testosterone (via PMFs, eurycoma, theanine, etc.).
- Then should come the *reinforcements* against episodes of stress in the form of a balanced adaptogen regimen.

RELAXATION AND CALMING SUPPLEMENTS

It is no surprise that dietary supplements marketed for promoting relaxation, reducing anxiety, and alleviating stress are among the top-selling products on the market. Millions of tired and stressed-out people (many of whom may be reading this book) can relate to promises of natural products that will enhance their brain function and make them feel better.

As discussed previously, physiologists and nutritionists regularly document the dramatic improvements in mood, emotions, confidence, and self-efficacy that result from some very simple lifestyle modifications. Regular exercise and adequate diet can result in profound changes in the body's own production of mood-elevating chemicals, such as the endorphins that cause "runner's high" and the neurotransmitters like serotonin that contribute to emotional well-being. In general terms, *any* amount of exercise can help to induce feelings of relaxation and calmness. Walking for twenty minutes on as many days of the week as possible (but at least three times per week) might be a good place to start.

On the nutritional side of things, it will probably come as no surprise that diet is intimately tied to emotions. Just think about your feelings as you contemplate gorging on that hot fudge sundae (weakness), followed by your feelings when you finally give in to the temptation (guilt) and start eating (elation), until you get to the bottom of the bowl (disappointment). All kidding aside, the foods we eat *directly* influence our moods, because the macronutrients (carbohydrates, proteins, fats) and micronutrients (vitamins, minerals, and phytonutrients) they contain ultimately act as potent neurochemicals. For example, a higher-protein diet can leave some people feeling energized, while a higher-carbohydrate diet can leave others feeling hungry, lethargic, and depressed.

For most people, the best advice for getting a handle on their emotional balance is to take a week or so to analyze how their diet affects their mood. Pay attention to every speck of food you eat and how it makes you feel. This is made easier by keeping a "food and mood" diary for seven to ten days, wherein you record every bite of food eaten (including quantities), time of day eaten, and mood and energy levels before and afterward. The patterns revealed in a food diary can be enlightening. But if the thought of adding such a task to your busy schedule stresses you out, then a less formal period of observation can be informative, too. Once you feel you know a bit about how certain foods influence your emotions, then you can decide where some of the dietary supplements outlined below may (or may not) fit into your lifestyle.

In very general terms, a number of popular herbs are used to help "take the edge off" after a particularly stressful day. Many of the herbs in this category are found in relaxing herbal teas and include chamomile, melissa, lemon balm, hops, oats, skullcap, and passionflower. Even though these herbs are widely used to help soothe ragged nerves (again, mostly as herbal teas), none of them have any strong or convincing scientific evidence to support their effectiveness against stress, anxiety, or elevated cortisol levels. This certainly doesn't mean they are useless—after all, a warm cup of tea can sometimes be just the thing to help reduce stress and bring you back to a more relaxed state.

Some of the more specific and effective dietary supplements for promoting relaxation include those listed in Table 8.6, and they are outlined in greater detail in the rest of this section. Many of these supplements are also used to treat mild forms of depression, anxiety, and insomnia, but they all have a general calming quality that can contribute to overall feelings of relaxation.

Table 8.6: Popular Antistress Supplements Frequently Used to Treat Depression, Anxiety, and Insomnia

Supplement	Dose (per Day)	Primary Effect
Kava kava	50–150 mg	Antianxiety
Melatonin	1–10 mg	Antianxiety/sleep aid
Valerian	250–500 mg	Antianxiety/sleep aid
Gotu kola	60–180 mg	Antianxiety
St. John's wort	450–900 mg	Relieves mild depression
5-HTP	300–900 mg	Relieves mild depression
SAM-e	200–600 mg	Relieves mild depression

Kava Kava

Kava (*Piper methysticum*) is a root from a pepper plant used for centuries by Pacific Islanders (e.g., Fijians and Hawaiians) as a ceremonial intoxicant to help people relax and socialize. Modern-day usage of kava is as a dietary supplement for relieving anxiety and tension. The active ingredients in kava, chemicals called *kavalactones*, act as a mild central nervous system depressant, but typically do not produce the hangover effects associated with alcohol.

Traditional preparation of the kava root involves cutting up freshly dug roots, chewing them, and then spitting them into a large communal bowl containing water or coconut milk. This unappetizing combination is then mixed, strained to remove any remaining large pieces, and passed around for everyone to share. It all sounds (and tastes!) pretty disgusting, but early Christian missionaries to the islands actually tried to ban kava parties because people were having such a good time preparing and passing the kava drinks. If you can't stomach the chewing and spitting part of kava preparation, the roots can be pounded until soft, then soaked in a fluid before drinking. The brew has a somewhat bitter taste and a slightly numbing or tingling sensation on the tongue.

Of course, kava is not very often prepared or consumed in the traditional way by average supplement users in the United States. Instead, the kava roots are dried and ground into a powder by machines. The powder can then be packed into capsules or tablets, blended into drinks, or dissolved in an alcohol-based extract. Americans spend about $30–$50 million annually on kava-containing products—a powerful testament to our high-stress lifestyles and our need for help in relaxing.

Although few well-designed studies have been conducted in the United States on kava in humans, several projects have been carried out in Europe. These trials have mostly been conducted in Germany, and have found kava (at a dose containing 50–150 mg per day of kavalactones) to be helpful in alleviating anxiety and other emotional problems related to stress. One study assessed various psychological stressors and found that after four weeks the group taking kava supplements showed significant decreases in stress in every category measured, in contrast to the placebo group, which showed little variation in any area.

No side effects or withdrawal symptoms have been noted during kava-supplementation studies or when people stopped taking the supplement, but recently several case studies have shown that kava supplementation may be linked to various forms of liver damage in some people. In light of these findings, some supplement companies are voluntarily removing their kava-containing products from the market. Additionally, the U.S. Food and Drug Administration in early 2002 issued a warning that kava carries a "potential risk" of causing severe liver damage and urged kava users and their doctors to be on the lookout for signs of liver injury. Therefore, until we know more about the potential liver toxicity associated with kava supplements, it would be prudent for people with liver damage to avoid kava and for healthy people to consume no more than 50 mg of kavalactones per day.

Because kava depresses the nervous system, it should not be taken with alcohol or in conjunction with antianxiety drugs. In addition, although kava appears to be helpful for alleviating cases of mild to moderate anxiety, self-medication with kava is probably not appropriate for individuals with major anxiety conditions. It is also advisable to refrain from using kava before driving. An interesting case occurred in Maryland a few years ago wherein a police officer pulled a man over for driving erratically. The man slurred his speech and had difficulty walking, so the officer reasonably assumed he was intoxicated, despite the man's insistence that he had not been drinking. Blood-alcohol measures indicated no alcohol in the man's system. After further questioning, it was discovered that the man had recently consumed several cups of kava tea.

Melatonin

Melatonin is a hormone produced in the pineal gland of the brain from the amino acid tryptophan. It is used in the body to help regulate sleep/wake cycles. Melatonin levels are lowest during midday and highest at night. Daylight is known to slow the production of melatonin, while darkness increases its production.

Dietary supplements containing melatonin promote relaxation and sleep, but the best evidence of its effectiveness comes from studies of people who have disturbed sleep/wake cycles, such as from jet lag and shift work. Several studies show that low-dose melatonin supplements (1–5 mg taken thirty to sixty minutes before bedtime) can help people sleep better, fall asleep faster, and have higher energy and alertness levels upon waking. Theoretical reasons also exist for melatonin's apparent benefits in alleviating depression, especially the type of depression brought on by a lack of sunlight during winter months and often referred to as *seasonal affective disorder* (SAD, also known as the "winter blues"). On the other hand, some studies suggest that melatonin can induce or deepen depression in susceptible individuals.

The interaction of melatonin with other supplements or drugs is unknown, but melatonin supplements may be dangerous for people with cardiovascular risks, due to the possibility of vasoconstriction and increased blood pressure. Additionally, the National Institutes of Health have warned about possible dangers of melatonin supplementation, including infertility, reduced sex drive in males, hypothermia, retinal damage, and interference with hormone replacement therapy. Information regarding the long-term effects of melatonin supplements is unavailable.

Melatonin can be viewed as a relatively inexpensive and nonaddictive alternative to over-the-counter chemical sleep aids. It may be particularly useful as a short-term regulator of sleep/wake cycles in cases such as getting the body clock back on schedule after crossing several time zones (jet lag). Studies of melatonin as a sleep aid or for relief of symptoms associated with jet lag have shown 1–10 mg to be effective, depending on the degree of sleep disturbance. Be careful, though, because the higher end of this dosage range can cause some people to experience vivid nightmares. High-dose melatonin supplements (around 50 mg) may disrupt female fertility and menstrual patterns and should be avoided except under the supervision of a reproductive physician.

Valerian

Valerian (*Valeriana officinalis*) has been used as a medicinal anti-anxiety herb and sleep aid since the days of the Romans. The dried roots of the plant are used in teas, tinctures, capsules, and tablets for promoting relaxation, inducing sleep, calming nerves, and reducing anxiety. It is unclear which of valerian's numerous compounds is the true active ingredient, but the combination of compounds appears to work together in the brain in a manner similar to the action of prescription tranquilizers such as Valium and Halcion. One problem, however, is that valerian is notoriously unstable; it loses its activity very quickly if it is not processed, packaged, and stored in exactly the right way.

Numerous studies in animals and humans support the effect of valerian as a mild sedative and sleep aid. In several studies, 400–600 mg of valerian extract, taken approximately one hour before bedtime, provides benefits in terms of overall relaxation, reduction of tension, and ability to fall asleep. Some products combine valerian with support herbs such as hops or melissa (lemon balm), both of which offer their own additional relaxation benefits with none of valerian's characteristic sweaty-sock odor.

Taken before bedtime, valerian appears to reduce the amount of time required to fall asleep. It is unknown, however, whether the quality of the sleep is affected by valerian consumption. Valerian is generally regarded as a mild tranquilizer and has been deemed safe by the German Commission E (the German regulatory body for herbal medicines) for treating "restlessness and sleeping disorders brought on by nervous conditions."

Because the activity and strength of valerian preparations can vary significantly from one product to the next, it is recommended whenever possible to select a standardized preparation containing 0.5–1.0 percent valerenic acids and to follow the package instructions for the particular product. As a general guideline, approximately 250–500 mg of a 5-to-1 or 6-to-1 extract can be taken before bed (as a sleep aid) or as needed as a mild tranquilizer.

Although valerian does not appear to be habit-forming or to

result in hangover-like morning drowsiness, it does seem to impair one's ability to concentrate for a few hours after taking it. Occasional reports of headaches and mild nausea are documented, but habituation or dependency is unlikely when it is used as directed. Valerian should be avoided by pregnant and lactating women, and by children. Individuals currently taking sedative drugs or antidepressant medications should consult with their personal physician before taking valerian, and no one should take the herb in conjunction with alcohol or other tranquilizers, or for a period of more than two weeks.

> *Mark,* the building contractor whom we met earlier, struggled with stress-related insomnia. Mark already got a great deal of physical activity at work, and because his wife (a fitness instructor) knew a lot about nutrition, he had help in eating a very well-balanced diet. He started on a supplement regimen that was targeted to control his cortisol levels and help him relax and sleep better. Mark's program included both theanine (100 mg taken with a bottle of water as he left the job site in the late afternoon) and valerian (250 mg taken thirty minutes before bedtime). The theanine helped him to relax without getting drowsy on his way home from work, and the valerian helped him to relax just a bit more and drop off to sleep faster. After only a few days on this regimen, Mark reported a deeper and more restful sleep than he had experienced in months. As a result of his better sleep quality, Mark's energy levels went up and his ability to concentrate at work was much improved.

Gotu Kola

Gotu kola *(Centella asiatica)* is an Indian herb that has been used for centuries in Ayurvedic (Indian) and traditional Chinese medicine to alleviate symptoms of depression and anxiety. Several animal studies have shown that gotu kola enhances performance in maze tests (which assess memory and learning ability as well as degree of anxiety) and reduces various symptoms of stress. Findings from human studies also suggest a beneficial effect of gotu kola in reducing anxiety and responses to laboratory-induced stress. It is interesting to note that a number of laboratory studies have also shown gotu kola to bind to specialized cellular receptors in the gastrointestinal tract called *cholecystokinin (CCK) receptors*. CCK receptors help regulate appetite, food intake, and eating behavior, and the binding of gotu kola to them may help modulate hunger and food cravings throughout the day, especially those cravings and urges for bingeing that can be brought on by stress. It is important to keep in mind that gotu kola should not be confused with the kola nut, which is completely unrelated and is often used in weight-loss and energy supplements as a natural source of caffeine.

In one investigation of the anxiolytic (antianxiety) effects of gotu kola, twenty healthy volunteers were given either a single 12-gram dose of gotu kola or a look-alike placebo. Results showed that compared with placebo, gotu kola significantly reduced the response of the subjects to a series of laboratory stressors (loud noises and other startling events) administered over the subsequent thirty to sixty minutes. Now, 12 grams is a pretty large dose of gotu kola, but the effect was quite fast and very powerful. Smaller doses are known to be effective in reducing stress response during the presence of normal, everyday stressors of the sort that most of us would encounter on a regular basis.

The activity of gotu kola has also been studied in another form of stress: that of injury. In animal studies, gotu kola extracts have been shown to increase the production of hydroxyproline and collagen, the structural components needed for wound healing, by 50–60 percent. Other studies have shown gotu kola to possess antioxidant effects that can be beneficial in wound healing, skin protection, and immune-system support. In these studies, the antioxidant effects of gotu kola, given twice daily for seven days, improved antioxidant capacity of the tissue by 35–75 percent and reduced free-radical damage by nearly 70 percent.

Gotu kola is frequently found in topical skin preparations for its benefits in speeding wound healing; dietary forms of the herb are generally provided in capsule or tablet form. Dietary intake of gotu kola appears to be nontoxic, but there is some anecdotal evidence that gotu kola may result in elevated blood-sugar levels, an effect that could be of concern to individuals with diabetes. Typical dosage recommendations are in the range of 60–180 mg per day of an extract standardized to contain 30–40 percent of the active triterpene compounds (asiaticoside, asiatic acid, and related compounds).

St. John's Wort

St. John's wort (*Hypericum perforatum*) is typically recommended as an herbal alternative to antidepressant medications. It is effective in balancing mood and lifting spirits, and in many people it is also quite beneficial in relieving the fatigue that is often associated with mild to moderate depression and high stress. People who are depressed or under constant stress often lack the energy to even get themselves out of bed in the morning, and their day is a never-ending battle against fatigue. By correcting neurotransmitter imbalances in the brain, St. John's wort can bring energy levels back to normal and help alleviate the crushing fatigue that accompanies depressed mood and chronic stress.

The precise active ingredients in St. John's wort are unknown, but extracts standardized to contain 0.3 percent hypericin and 3 percent hyperforin, in doses of 900 mg per day, are known to be effective in alleviating mild to moderate depressive symptoms. St. John's wort is readily available as capsules containing the standardized extract. Using these hypericin/hyperforin extracts, numerous clinical studies have shown that people with mild or moderate depression tend to respond to St. John's wort to about the same degree as they would to some of the older prescription antidepressant medications, with fewer side effects. A number of well-controlled studies comparing the St. John's wort extract to prescription antidepressants such as fluoxetine (Prozac), sertraline (Zoloft), and paroxetine (Paxil) have found St. John's wort to be comparable in effectiveness, but superior to prescription drugs with regard to tolerability. Overall, more than a dozen double-blind placebo-controlled studies have been conducted—albeit mostly small ones—and the majority support the case for the effectiveness of St. John's wort in alleviating mild to moderate depression, but not severe depression.

St. John's wort is quite safe in terms of observed side effects, the most common of which are mild gastrointestinal upset, mild allergic reactions (skin rash), and insomnia/restlessness, usually when taken close to bedtime. There have been no published reports of serious adverse side effects from taking the herb alone, and animal studies using large doses of St. John's wort have not shown any serious problems. The most commonly studied adverse effect of St. John's wort is its ability to cause photosensitivity in fair-skinned individuals, increasing their risk of sunburn.

Although direct side effects from consuming St. John's wort appear to be quite rare, several recent reports have raised the possibility that the herb may interact with and decrease the effectiveness of various medications, including HIV drugs (protease inhibitors), immunosuppressants (such as cyclosporin for organ transplants), digoxin (for congestive heart failure), blood thinners (Coumadin/warfarin), chemotherapy drugs (olanzapine/clozapine), and asthma medications (theophylline). If you are currently taking any of these drugs or other prescription medications, *discontinue taking or do not begin taking St. John's wort* without first consulting your personal physician. Abrupt withdrawal of the herb could increase blood levels of various medications, which could be dangerous in certain cases.

St. John's wort appears to be helpful in about 50 to 60 percent of cases, but as with prescription antidepressants, the full effect takes about four to six weeks to develop. It is important to note that St. John's wort should *never* be used for the treatment of severe depression (feelings of suicide, extreme inability to cope with daily life, severe anxiety, or extreme fatigue); in such cases, physician-directed drug therapy may mean the difference between life and death.

5-HTP

5-HTP (5-hydroxytryptophan) is a derivative of the amino acid tryptophan. In the body, tryptophan is converted into 5-HTP, which can then be converted into serotonin, a potent neurotransmitter in the brain. Although 5-HTP is not found at any significant level in a normal diet, tryptophan is found in a wide variety of protein foods. The 5-HTP used in dietary supplements is derived from the seeds of an African plant, *Griffonia simplicifolia,* and is typically used as a treatment for relieving mild depression, counteracting insomnia, promoting weight loss, and reducing overall sensations of stress and pain, such as migraine headaches, fibromyalgia, and general muscle pain.

5-HTP is typically used to treat mild depression and to combat stress, and this is done based on the theory that as a precursor to serotonin, supplements of 5-HTP can increase serotonin levels and influence mood, sleep patterns, and pain control. In a few small studies, 5-HTP has been shown to be as effective as prescription antidepressant medications—and with fewer side effects. In other studies, doses of 5-HTP in the range of 300–900 mg per day have resulted in benefits in reducing pain associated with migraines and fibromyalgia, reducing appetite, and promoting sleep, possibly by increasing blood and brain levels of serotonin. It appears that there are "responders," individuals who experience an elevation in 5-HTP levels in the blood, as well as "nonresponders," who see no such increase.

The most significant safety concern related to 5-HTP supplements is the remote possibility for contamination with a compound linked to a disorder known as *eosinophilic myalgia syndrome* (EMS), which results in muscle pain and weakness, vomiting, headache, and, in rare cases, death. In 1989 an outbreak of EMS was linked to contaminated tryptophan supplements—not to the tryptophan per se, but to a contaminant in the supplements. As a result, the FDA banned the sale of all tryptophan supplements, a move that has been widely criticized by people on both sides of the supplement debate. The banned tryptophan supplements were manufactured from a bacterial source in a fermentation process, whereas 5-HTP is extracted from the seeds of a plant—so it is less likely (though not impossible) that the contaminant associated with EMS, commonly known as *peak X,* is present in 5-HTP supplements. Some supplement manufacturers and raw-material suppliers conduct quality-control tests to confirm the absence of peak X in their 5-HTP supplements. If you decide to try 5-HTP, it is suggested that you contact the manufacturer of your supplement for confirmation that their products have passed this type of analysis. Supplemental forms of 5-HTP are available in capsule or tablet form, as extracts from griffonia seeds (providing 15–20 percent 5-HTP), and in synthetic form (99 percent pure).

In addition to the above safety considerations, 5-HTP supplements are not recommended for children or for women who are pregnant or lactating. People currently taking prescription antidepressants, weight-control medications, or herbal remedies for depression (such as St. John's wort) should not combine these treatments with 5-HTP supplements, except on the advice and guidance of a nutritionally oriented physician.

SAM-e

S-adenosylmethionine (SAM-e) is a form of the sulfur-containing amino acid methionine, combined with adenosine (part of the energy compound ATP). Like methionine, SAM-e is involved in numerous metabolic processes in the body that require sulfur—such as the methylation reactions. The body typically manufactures all the SAM-e it requires from methionine consumed in protein foods, but a defect in methylation or a deficiency in any of the cofactors required for SAM-e production (such as methionine, choline, or the B vitamins) is theorized to reduce the body's ability to produce SAM-e.

It has been hypothesized that a defect in the body's methylation process is central to the biochemical basis of certain neuropsychiatric disorders, and that chronic stress can interfere with the body's ability to conduct these methylation reactions. Tissue levels of SAM-e have been found to be low in the elderly and in patients suffering from depression and chronic stress. SAM-e has performed as well as conventional antidepressant drugs in studies of depression, probably due to an increase in brain levels of neurotransmitters such as serotonin and dopamine.

SAM-e is quite safe at recommended doses and has the distinct advantage over some other herbal medicines of being a naturally occurring compound in the body, which suggests that supplementation with SAM-e simply provides an additional dietary source of this nutrient. Other antidepressant compounds that are available as dietary supplements, such as St. John's wort, could be viewed as more of a pharmacological approach to relieving depression because they are not naturally found in the body. The problem with dietary supplements containing SAM-e is their cost—SAM-e is an expensive ingredient. The good news, however, is that the mood benefits of SAM-e are more affordable (delivered at 200–600 mg per day) than the joint-health benefits of the supplement (for which you'd need 1,200–1,400 mg per day). Even at 200–600 mg per day, however, SAM-e tablets (the most stable form) generally cost $20 to $30 for a ten-day supply.

SUMMARY: RELAXATION SUPPLEMENTS

So where do these calming herbs fit in? They can certainly represent an effective approach to promoting relaxation and de-stressing a person during periods of particularly high stress. However, when it comes to designing your specific cortisol-control regimen, it may be helpful to take it step-by-step (see the boxed text on the next page). As such, most of the supplements covered in this section should be thought of as secondary choices to be used in specific cases of depression, insomnia, or when something is needed to take the edge off after a particularly stressful day.

We've now covered the five most important steps for controlling stress and modulating cortisol levels by taking supplements:

1. Avoid excessive doses of supplements that can increase cortisol levels (stimulants such as ephedra and caffeine)

2. Take a multivitamin/multimineral supplement as a cortisol-control foundation

3. Focus on targeted modulation of cortisol, testosterone, and HSD, especially during periods of high stress

4. Consider adding "reinforcement" supplements against stress in the form of adaptogens

5. Use calming supplements to fight depression, insomnia, and frazzled nerves

Stressed Jess will have to follow each of these five steps for optimal cortisol control, with a particular emphasis on the third step.

Strained Jane may be able to get away with following only steps 1–3; she may never have a need to progress to steps 4 and 5.

Relaxed Jack, as laid-back as he appears, he can also benefit from following the first two steps on a regular basis, but he may need to progress to step 3 during his occasional high-stress periods.

Faced with all of these recommendations, it is logical that you may feel a bit confused about how to put them into practice—but don't stress out about it! The next, and final, chapter pulls all of the preceding chapters together into the simple plan, summarized in Chapter 7, called the SENSE Lifestyle Program.

· · · · · · · · · · · ·
· · ·
· ·
·

CHAPTER 9

Putting It All Together: The SENSE Lifestyle Program

You've heard it before—the familiar message that health experts (including your dear old grandmother) have been repeating for years: Get enough sleep, eat right, and exercise. Yes, it's a tired old mantra, but these three steps are probably the most effective tools available for combating stress and keeping cortisol levels from getting the best of us. Stress researchers from Yale to the University of California have shown over and over that the best way to manage stress, from both a physical and a psychological perspective, is to adhere to the basic tenets of good health promotion—eat right, sleep, and exercise. (See how smart your grandma was?) Failure to do so, as we know by now, causes an elevation in cortisol levels and sets the stage for chronic diseases.

Unfortunately, when we are exposed to periods of heightened stress, what do we do? We do exactly the *opposite* of what we're supposed to. Instead of exercising, we stop our workout program, because stress makes us feel as if we simply don't have enough time. Instead of eating sensibly, we allow our cortisol levels to become elevated, which makes us hungryand therefore more likely to grab something at the drive-through window. And instead of getting enough sleep to help our bodies counteract the debilitating effects of stress, we stay up late, wake up early, and suffer from restlessness and insomnia.

As a nutritionist, physiologist, and lifestyle coach for more than a decade, I have used the concepts outlined in *The Cortisol Connection* to help thousands of clients optimize their own metabolic profiles—and achieve the lasting weight loss they have been looking for. More often than not, these are people who have tried other diets and have lost weight, but who have had that weight come right back (often with a bit more, as an added "bonus"). Like many of my clients, you may already be following what could be viewed as an excellent diet and exercise plan—but no matter how many calories you cut or how many minutes you exercise, you just can't seem to shed those last few pounds. Sound familiar?

BE THE BALLOON:
THE "3S" APPROACH TO MANAGING
METABOLIC ADAPTATION

When I teach metabolic concepts to participants in our SENSE Lifestyle Program I often use a balloon to illustrate the concept of *metabolic adaptation*. I point out that balloons come in a variety of shapes and sizes (just like our bodies), and when we influence one aspect of metabolism (as illustrated by pushing in on the right side of the balloon), we get an opposite reaction in another aspect of metabolism (the balloon swells on its left side). Physicists would refer to this concept as Newton's Third Law of Motion (every action has an equal and opposite reaction), but nutritionists refer to it as metabolic adaptation, and it is one of the overarching reasons why lasting weight loss is so difficult to achieve—unless you know precisely how to use diet and exercise to guide your metabolism in the right direction.

The classic example of how metabolic adaptation applies to weight loss is the one that we've been discussing throughout this book, in which you cut calories to lose weight, but at the same time your resting metabolic rate (RMR, the number of calories your body burns at rest) also drops—so weight loss continues for a few days or weeks, and then it stops (the dreaded weight-loss "plateau"). The weight may even start to creep back on to your hips and belly. This is an example of your body's adapting its metabolism (by burning fewer calories) to its new environment (fewer calories being consumed, higher cortisol levels, lower testosterone levels, etc.)—and while the process may have been advantageous for our ancestors' survival when they faced starvation, it doesn't exactly help our weight-loss efforts in the twenty-first century.

The key to lasting weight-loss success is to "outsmart" your body's own process of metabolic adaptation. In other words, you not only need to *think* about the balloon, you need to *be* the balloon! You need to use what I call the "3S" approach, which calls for small, simultaneous, and sustained changes in metabolism to help you achieve long-term weight-loss success. The 3S approach is fully incorporated into SENSE, and it means that you control metabolism *just enough* to achieve a desired effect (weight loss) but not so much that you cross the line into metabolic adaptation.

By *small*, I mean that we avoid extreme or "big" changes in metabolism, because extreme changes set off an almost immediate adaptation that causes our bodies to conserve energy and slow weight loss. Small changes help us to keep "shrinking our balloon"—and most of us want to be smaller balloons.

By *simultaneous*, I mean that we need to influence several different aspects of metabolism at the same time, including cortisol, testosterone, and HSD—which in turn help to modulate other hormones and other aspects of the enzyme system such as insulin/blood sugar, growth hormone, thyroid hormones, serotonin, norepinephrine, and others that I collectively refer to as *metabolic control points* (MCPs). A significant problem with many popular diets is their inappropriate focus on a single aspect of metabolism—such as appetite control or calorie intake. These are both certainly important facets of any successful weight-loss regimen, but when your diet focuses too much on a single aspect of metabolism, it is very easy for your body to adapt to maintain your existing weight. By contrast, it is much more difficult for your body to fully adapt to small changes made simultaneously in several areas of metabolism.

Finally, by *sustained*, I mean that we need to keep at it. Sometimes this entails changing the plan slightly from time to time in order to stay one step ahead of our own metabolic adaptation. The good news is that the small/simultaneous approach to metabolic control is quite easy to sustain—for life. In fact, most of my clients wouldn't go back to their "old" weight-maintenance approaches if I paid them to do so. Why? Simple. Because by following the principles outlined in SENSE, they look great and they feel great—and who would want to change that?

Researchers at the National Institutes of Health (NIH) have been studying the behavioral effects of heightened stress for more than thirty years. Their work shows quite clearly that stress causes us to undereat during the early stages of our stress response (maybe up to an hour), while our longer-term response to chronic stress, lasting from hours to days, is to overeat. This effect was confirmed in weight-loss centers around the country and the world after the September 11, 2001, terrorist attacks on the World Trade Center and the Pentagon. The resulting stress led many dieters to report stress-induced suppression of appetite, caused by feeling sick to their stomachs, followed some hours later by stress-induced food binges, caused by a cortisol-stimulated appetite. NIH researchers have estimated that at least one-quarter of all Americans—more than sixty million people—will suffer (or already have suffered) an abnormal stress response to the events of September 11, which sets many of us up for increased risk of chronic diseases such as obesity, diabetes, heart disease, and others.

Enough doom and gloom. We know that stress is "bad" and we know that chronically elevated cortisol levels are "bad"—but what can we do about it? That's where the SENSE program comes into play. SENSE, as you know by now, stands for stress management, exercise, nutrition, supplementation, and evaluation. With SENSE, you'll eat all of the foods you love, but you'll learn how to use your food consumption to control the effects of cortisol, testosterone, HSD, and other MCPs in your body—and ultimately to control how many calories you burn off or store as fat. A special feature of this final chapter is its practical approach to helping you make SENSE a part of your everyday life.

STRESS MANAGEMENT

As mentioned throughout the book, a variety of effective stress-management techniques exist that can be very helpful in controlling one's bodily responses to stressful situations. It is not, however, the focus of this book to highlight any specific stress-management technique—for that, there are many excellent sources, a few of which are listed in the Resources section. For a handful of quick stress-management tips that don't require major lifestyle change and that are easy enough to begin incorporating into your life today, you can also review the list I've provided in Chapter 7.

I have broken the entire category of stress management into three simple categories: (1) avoid stress, (2) manage stress, and (3) get enough sleep. To some readers, this may appear to be an overly simplistic approach to a topic as complex as stress management. Those readers are quite correct—it *is* simplistic—but for the vast majority of people (your author included), these three simple steps will provide the greatest return for the time they are prepared to devote to the specific practice of stress management (which is not a great deal of time). At this point, let's recap some ideas presented in Chapter 7 for managing stress, as well as throw in a few new ones.

Avoid Stress (Whenever You Can)

It probably comes as no surprise that the most effective stress-management technique is to simply avoid all the stressful situations that you encounter in the first place. If you do this, you have no exposure to stress, no overactive stress response, and no increase in cortisol levels. Obviously, the goal of avoiding *all* stressful situations is unrealistic, but with proper planning it may be possible to avoid *some* of them—or at least to plan effective strategies for dealing with the situations that cause you the most stress.

As an example, one of the things that causes me a great deal of stress is sitting in traffic. My personal strategy to avoid this source of stress is to make sure I stay ahead of the traffic by leaving the house as early as possible in the morning and leaving the office as early as possible in the evening. Of course, with two small children at home, it is often impossible to leave the house as early as planned, nor does the pile of work on my desk always allow me to leave the office as early as I wish. On these days, when my first-line stress-avoidance strategy of leaving early fails, I know I'll be sitting in traffic and I know I'll need to employ my backup plan, which is to listen to a book on tape. The book on tape allows me to avoid a personal source of stress because it enables me either to learn something new or to lose myself in a story—instead of stewing my way through a time-wasting traffic jam.

It is important to understand that each person will have a different strategy for avoiding their own personal stressors; the key is to find the plan (and a backup plan) that works best for you.

Manage Stress (As Effectively As You Can)

Obviously, if you can't avoid stress, then you've got to manage stress as effectively as possible. It might be instructive to review the discussion in Chapter 7 about the three mediating factors in the body's response to stress: whether there is any *outlet* for the stress, whether the stressor is *predictable*, and whether the individual thinks they have any *control* over the stressor.

Meditation, yoga, or getting in touch with your "inner self" may all be perfectly acceptable and beneficial outlets for stress, but managing stress is a very individualized concept, and a technique that reduces stress for one person may very well increase it for another. Readers who want to go beyond the approaches to stress management covered in this book are referred to the Resources section for a list of books that focus on a more emotional or psychological approach to stress management.

Get Some Sleep!

Yes, you say, it makes perfect sense that you need to spend enough time in bed when you're stressed; unfortunately, stress also throws a great, big monkey wrench into your normal sleep patterns. Not to mention the fact that our modern, Type C lifestyles have us living "24/7" schedules—so who's got time to sleep anyway? The main problem with this situation is that, aside from the well-known bad mood and inability to concentrate that we've all experienced from too few hours in the sack, sleep researchers have recently linked a chronic lack of sleep to problems with blood-sugar control, increased appetite, and a higher risk of diabetes and obesity—and chronically elevated cortisol is the obvious culprit. Researchers at both the University of Pennsylvania and the University of Chicago have shown that while too little sleep (six hours per night for a week) heightens an already revved-up stress response and keeps cortisol levels elevated, getting back into a more normal sleep pattern (eight hours per night) can reverse many of these detrimental changes and bring cortisol levels back to normal.

Getting more sleep, of course, is easier said than done, so the experts at the National Sleep Foundation recommend a few simple steps, like the ones listed below, for helping to get a person back onto track for obtaining the eight hours of sleep that most of us need each night:

- Establish a regular bedtime and a regular wake-up time—and stick to them for one week, even on the weekends (no matter how hard it is for the first few days). Sleep researchers tell us that within the time span of one week our body clocks will reset themselves to the new schedule.

- Do something calming in the hour or so before bedtime—such as relaxing with a book and a cup of warm chamomile tea, doing a crossword puzzle, or whatever else provides you with a few moments of peaceful reflection. My own getting-ready-for-bed ritual typically also includes a

100 mg dose of theanine (thirty to sixty minutes before I plan to climb under the covers), some light reading, and a background of low-key jazz music from the local public-radio station.

- Avoid exercise within three hours of bedtime. Exercise causes an increase in hormones, body temperature, and alertness—each of which will thwart efforts to fall asleep. For most people, exercising after work or even right after dinner (between 5:00 P.M. and 7:00 P.M.) is probably okay (assuming bedtime will be three to four hours later), because sufficient time is still available to allow the body to calm down and return to resting levels.

EXERCISE

Like getting enough sleep during stressful periods, getting enough exercise is another one of those no-brainers—but few of us follow through on what we know we should be doing. Ideally we've all experienced that feeling of postexercise relaxation that comes from elevated endorphins and lowered stress hormones. Aside from the feel-good, mind-clearing effects of exercise, however, are the obvious general health benefits for the heart and muscles, and also the general antistress benefits that help to control appetite, regulate blood sugar, curb overeating, and improve sleep.

The high-stress/low-sleep/no-exercise cycle is a vicious one—but breaking it, even by doing a small amount of exercise several days a week, can yield dramatic benefits. The key point here is that you don't need to become an Ironman triathlete or start training for a marathon. A simple game of racquetball, a walk around the block, or a quick circuit of sit-ups and push-ups before you head out the door to work will go a long way toward getting those cortisol levels back into a healthy range. Even light physical activity in small, manageable doses will trigger a cascade of stress-busting benefits, from lowering blood pressure to improving mood.

Exercise and Diet as a Fountain of Youth

As we age, our metabolic rate drops, and most of us begin to pack on the pounds. If, in response to stress, we add fat in our abdominal area, our body shape changes from one resembling an hourglass to one more resembling a shot glass—and repeated diets only compound the problem.

Recall from Chapter 6 that most of us will experience a drop in metabolism of about 0.5 percent per year after the age of twenty. This phenomenon is largely due to a loss of about five to ten pounds of muscle tissue every decade—and that often translates into your fifty-year-old body carrying around thirty extra pounds of fat compared to when you were twenty! And this result specifically comes from a slight decline in your metabolic rate.

Many people attempt to eat "right" and follow a regular exercise program, and yet they still seem to gain weight. One of the reasons for this may be a change in their thermogenic potential (their ability to burn sufficient calories) because of some small (but important) dietary choices. For example, researchers at the University of Massachusetts have shown that certain dietary patterns, such as eating one or more midday snacks, are associated with a reduced risk of obesity (39 percent reduction in the case of healthy snacking), while other dietary habits, such as skipping breakfast, can increase obesity risk (450 percent increase in obesity risk from skipping breakfast). The dramatic difference here is largely due to a change in metabolic rate (snacking increases it, while skipping breakfast reduces it)—so dietary patterns that encourage a greater expenditure of calories are also those that tend to result in a lower body weight over time. In the case of breakfast, even our grandmothers told us that it is the "most important meal of the day," and when it comes to dieting you should consider breakfast a "free" meal! This is because eating breakfast increases your metabolic rate by 100–200 calories—while skipping breakfast slows down your metabolism by about the same amount. This means that by skipping breakfast (as compared to eating it), the overall difference balances out at 200–400 calories of lost calorie burning (thus the whopping 450 percent increase in obesity risk noted by the University of Massachusetts researchers).

Before we continue with our discussion of ways to enhance thermogenesis, let's consider a few guidelines that everyone who's attempting to lose weight should be aware of:

Caution: Calorie restriction will reduce your overall metabolic rate.

Acute calorie restriction typically causes a sharp decline in body temperature and the number of calories that you'll burn in a given day. By spacing appropriate meals and snacks throughout the day, and eating them in the right proportions (see below), you'll balance calorie levels to counteract this drop in metabolic rate.

Caution: Dehydration will reduce your thermogenic potential.

Drink plenty of water! Water is an important catalyst for weight loss because proper hydration is essential for fat burning, maintenance of muscle mass, and boosting overall metabolism. If you're dehydrated, even to a slight degree, your cortisol levels will rise and your metabolic rate will drop. Your hydration needs vary based on environmental conditions and exercise levels, but the basic rule of thumb to drink eight glasses of water each day is a good one. This rule is based upon a chemical estimate of how much water is needed to metabolize 1,500–2,000 calories from a mixed diet.

Where Does Exercise Fit In?

Remember from earlier sections that the key benefit of exercise for weight control is *not* that it burns a significant number of calories. Exercise certainly burns some calories, but far fewer than you may think. Instead, the primary value of exercise as part of a weight-control regimen lies in its profound effects on modulating levels of cortisol, testosterone, growth hormone, serotonin, and metabolic rate (with cortisol and serotonin control being responsible for many of the "feel good" effects of a workout).

The metabolic benefits of exercise are far-reaching, but from a weight-control perspective, a regular exercise program "teaches" our muscles to transport glucose more efficiently and to respond to cortisol more effectively. Exercise also improves our body's sensitivity to both insulin and cortisol, so we are able to get by with much lower levels of both of these powerful metabolic hormones and therefore avoid many of the health problems (such as weight gain) that are associated with chronically elevated levels.

An interesting side effect of optimizing your cortisol levels is an increase both in general caloric expenditure and in specific burning of fat (otherwise known as thermogenesis). This means that exercise *on its own* will influence, to a certain degree, each of the primary metabolic control points (MCPs) related to body-weight regulation—so get out there and do it.

Regular exercise is often promoted as a tool for preventing weight gain, and there is good evidence that people who are more active have a reduced risk of gaining weight. One study from the School of Public Health at Harvard University followed a large group of men over two years. At the beginning of the study, the most active men and those who watched fewer hours of television were less likely to be overweight, and after two years those who were most active and who watched fewer hours of television had gained less weight. Data from several national surveys (in both the United States and other countries) clearly show that people who maintain higher levels of physical activity are less likely to gain weight, or at least tend to gain less weight than their inactive counterparts.

Overall, then, whether exercise is a good tool for promoting weight *loss* is controversial. A number of recent scientific reviews of studies related to the effect of physical activity on weight loss concluded that adding exercise to a reduced-calorie diet only leads to modest additional weight loss (five to seven pounds over several months), but that regular exercise is strongly associated with *maintenance* of weight loss. Therefore, although exercise may be a less important tool for initial weight loss than calorie reduction, it is an important factor in the prevention of weight regain.

So, with most of the available evidence suggesting that physical activity plays a more important role in reducing age-related weight gain than it does in actually promoting weight loss, the obvious question is "Why isn't exercise more effective in promoting weight loss?" The answer is because it is simply very difficult to promote a substantial negative energy balance with exercise. Negative energy balance is the state where a person expends more energy (calories) than he or she consumes. To achieve a state of negative energy balance, one must consume fewer calories, expend more energy, or both. This seems like a pretty simple task, but the reality is that most adult Americans lack a good understanding of the energy value of different foods and exercises. Most people, including professional dieticians and physiologists, tend to underestimate the caloric value of food and overestimate the caloric value of exercise. Consider some of the values in the table below:

The Energy Cost of Exercise Versus Diet

Energy (Calories)*	Exercise for 30 Minutes	Dietary Equivalent
100	Walking, leisurely pace	¾ cup ice cream
150	Walking, brisk pace	6 Oreo cookies
200	Stationary cycling, easy	3 Tbsp. peanut butter
240	Lap swimming, leisurely	20 potato chips
240	Aerobic exercise class	1 slice pizza
300	Lap swimming, vigorous	12 Hershey Kisses
300	Stationary cycling, vigorous	1 fried chicken leg
300	Running, slow pace	1 Burger King cheese-burger
500	Running, fast pace	Taco Bell bean burrito with cheese

* Estimate based on a person who weighs 175 pounds. For a person who weighs more than 175 pounds, the estimated energy expenditure is slightly higher, and for someone who weighs less than 175 pounds, it's slightly lower.

As you can see, it is easy to wipe out the calories burned off by exercise with a few bites of the wrong foods. With a caloric deficit of thirty-five hundred calories needed to lose one pound of fat, and a general goal to lose about one pound of pure fat per week (with no loss of muscle), this would require a caloric deficit of five hundred to one thousand calories *each day*. For most people, this would mean thirty to sixty minutes of *intense* exercise daily (which I'd love to see more people doing)—but since most American adults are extremely sedentary and since about 40 percent get *no* physical activity, this level of exercise would be difficult to adhere to for most people.

In one study from the University of Pennsylvania, women who had lost weight were followed over the subsequent twelve months. The threshold level of exercise needed to prevent weight regain corresponded to approximately eighty minutes of brisk walking per day. The people enrolled in the National Weight Control Registry (NWCR) report a similar level of activity. (The NWCR is a large database of individuals who have maintained a minimum thirty-pound weight loss for at least one year.) In addition, recent data from researchers in Japan, Colorado, and Massachusetts suggest that accumulating twelve thousand to sixteen thousand steps per day (measured with pedometers) can really help one to prevent weight regain.

What Type of Exercise Should You Do?

Any type of exercise will work—as long as you do it! You simply need to get out there and move your body for at least three to six hours each week (thirty to sixty minutes per day, six days a week). If our goal were simply to burn as many calories as possible with exercise, then we'd be shooting for as much intensity as we could stand (exercising as hard as possible for as many minutes as we could).

If you're "too busy" to exercise (the most common excuse for not exercising), then you need to accept the fact that you will never lose those last twenty pounds, because without exercise your metabolic control of blood sugar and cortisol will never be optimized.

Think about all the things in which you invest thirty to sixty minutes each day—television, newspapers, Internet surfing, etc.—and then ask yourself if investing that same amount of time in your health, in your body, and in yourself is worth it. I think we both know what the answer will be.

The exercise recommendations that we follow as part of the SENSE program attempt to maximize the most metabolic benefits within the shortest time commitment possible. This is because most people do not have a lot of time in their stressful lives to devote to exercise. For this reason, we utilize a three-times-weekly regimen of interval training (either running or walking). After a five- to ten-minute warm-up, the exercise alternates between high- and low-intensity levels as follows:

1 minute high intensity / 1 minute low intensity*

2 minutes high intensity / 2 minutes low intensity

3 minutes high intensity / 3 minutes low intensity

2 minutes high intensity / 2 minutes low intensity

1 minute high intensity / 1 minute low intensity

* Note that the intensity levels will be relative to your individual fitness level. A general guideline is that "high" intensity is not an "all-out effort" but rather a level that gets you breathing hard enough that you have difficulty carrying on a conversation with your exercise buddy. The "low" intensity intervals are easy enough to allow full recovery before your next hard interval—and also easy enough for you to talk without getting out of breath.

These eighteen minutes of interval training are followed by five to ten minutes of easy cool-down exercise—for a total duration of about thirty minutes. Compared to exercising at a "steady moderate" pace for this same thirty-minute period, the interval approach will burn more than double the number of calories (401 versus 189) and will result in better control of cortisol, testosterone, and growth hormone.

Many of our participants use walking as their primary form of exercise—and we encourage them to walk as fast as they can. The faster you walk, the more calories you burn. For example, a sixty-minute walk at three miles per hour (twenty minutes to cover each mile) burns about 240 calories (for a 150-pound person)—but speeding up to four miles per hour (fifteen minutes/mile) burns that many calories in about forty minutes. Walking at five miles per hour (which is a pretty fast twelve-minute mile) burns even more calories.

Follow this regimen for three to five days each week for a year, and you're burning off about ten pounds of pure fat. In our SENSE program, we encourage walking whenever possible. If you find it tough to maintain a fast walking pace, try doing short intervals of faster walking (maybe for a minute) followed by periods of slower walking. A popular workout for our participants (similar to the interval regimen above) is to walk for thirty minutes and to alternate one minute of fast walking with four minutes of moderate walking for the entire half hour (e.g., walk at a moderate pace for four minutes, then speed it up for one minute, then go back to your moderate pace for four minutes, and then go back up to the faster one for one minute—repeat).

See the Resources section for some excellent ideas to get you started on a regular stress-busting exercise program, and also review the list below to jump-start your thinking about ways to sneak small increments of exercise into your daily routine:

- At the mall or grocery store, add a few hundred yards of walking to your daily activity tally by parking in the middle or back of the lot instead of at the front.

- If you use public transportation, try riding your bike to the train station or bus stop, or park your car a few blocks away and walk the rest of the way to catch your ride.

- At the airport, be a rebel and take the stairs instead of the escalator (be sure to smile at the people on the escalator; you'll feel better just by doing that).

- Put a basket on the front of your bicycle. You might look like Mary Poppins, but now you can use the bike to run short errands to the store.

- Instead of having a neighborhood kid (or your own kids) do your exercise for you, get out there yourself to mow the lawn, sweep the steps, rake the leaves, and shovel the driveway.

Kristen was about as Type C (high cortisol) as anyone you could imagine. An honor student and champion distance runner during her college years, she now worked for a large hospital group as a director of nursing. Among her fellow nurses, Kristen was notorious for putting in long hours, taking paperwork home with her, and being on call at all hours of the day and night. Kristen considered herself to have a "high-energy" personality; she felt she thrived on the demands and stress that came with managing a large department.

For six years Kristen did just fine. Despite the high-stress work that followed her home, and despite having chronically elevated cortisol levels from that high stress—as well as from inadequate sleep and a poor diet—she seemed to be able to handle her stress load perfectly well. She was promoted several times at work, maintained her athletic figure and healthy body weight from college, and enjoyed a loving relationship with her former college boyfriend, and now husband, Jim.

Everything in Kristen's life was going according to plan—everything was perfect—and then all hell broke loose. The straw that broke the camel's back, so to speak, was the birth of Kristen's first child. Having a baby was something that both Kristen and Jim had been planning and looking forward to since before they were married, so they were both well prepared mentally for the arrival of their new bundle of joy. The problem, however, was that Kristen was trying to maintain her prebaby work schedule along with her new motherhood duties. Jim helped with the baby as much as possible, but his travel schedule as a district sales manager meant that he was out of town on business at least a few times each month, leaving Kristen to juggle work, day care, and nightly feedings for the baby. The combination of this being Kristen's first baby and her self-described tendency to be a "worrier" (about the baby, about her work, and about Jim when he was traveling) caused her to experience some of the highest stress levels—and highest cortisol levels—of her entire life. Couple these high stress levels with changes in her exercise program (rarely having the time) and in her diet (grabbing whatever junk food happened to be most convenient), and Kristen was on a crash course with cortisol.

Kristen's elevated cortisol levels manifested themselves primarily in the form of an inability to lose the "baby weight" she had gained during pregnancy, a growing struggle to stay focused on the complex tasks required of her at work, and great difficulty in falling asleep at night and then in getting back to sleep after waking with the baby.

Kristen started following the SENSE program with the primary goal of using it as a structure to control her diet and lose the excess pregnancy weight. As a former competitive athlete, she knew the importance of regular exercise for general health, but with the demands placed on her at home and work, there simply were not enough hours in the day to schedule what Kristen considered to be a worthwhile amount of exercise. Her idea of worthwhile exercise was to drive fifteen minutes to the gym, participate in a forty-five-minute high-intensity aerobic-dance class, stretch, shower, and then drive home. This ideal exercise program would have taken almost two hours out of her day. No wonder she had no time for exercise.

The first step, when it came to incorporating some exercise (the first E in SENSE) into her daily routine, was to get her to think about exercise in a different way. Over the next several weeks, Kristen began to sprinkle small amounts of exercise throughout the day—taking the stairs whenever possible at work, pushing her baby in his stroller when the weather was nice, and parking her car at the back of the parking lot and walking the hundred yards to the front door of the grocery store. Kristen even took her sprinkling of exercise to the extreme by performing a set of deep knee bends while her baby was swallowing between each spoonful of baby food. Suffice it to say, Kristen embraced the concept of sneaking exercise into her day—and even though she would have preferred to be out running five miles or sweating at the gym, she accepted the fact that this was as good as it was going to get at this point in her life.

In terms of nutrition, Kristen's greatest challenge was her constant snacking. Because she had difficulty planning the balanced meals she knew she should be eating, she was in a constant state of "grab and go"—and there didn't appear to be any solution for changing that pattern. Instead, the most practical strategy for Kristen was to make each of the "grab and go" meals a more balanced blend of carbohydrates, proteins, fats, fiber, vitamins, and minerals. A logical way to do this was to incorporate meal replacements; that is, shakes and energy bars. For Kristen, grabbing a shake for breakfast or a bar for the drive to work offered just the right amount of structure. Doing so enabled her to get the fuel she needed to keep her metabolism humming, it helped her control her blood sugar and banished her late-afternoon cravings for sweets, and it gave her the willpower she needed to resist sneaking to the fridge for a late-night snack after putting the baby to bed.

Perhaps the aspect of SENSE that made the most significant impact on Kristen's stress and cortisol levels was her incorporation of dietary supplements into her daily schedule. During her pregnancy she had already become accustomed to taking a daily multivitamin, so it was easy for her to continue this positive habit. In addition to her multi, Kristen also added a twice-daily theanine supplement (50 mg with breakfast and 100 mg before bed) and a midday dose of *Cordyceps sinensis* and American ginseng. The combination of cordyceps and ginseng provided the dual benefits of blood-sugar regulation (and added appetite control) plus an energy boost, without the side effects of stimulants. Theanine helped Kristen to stay calm and focused during the day (without drowsiness), while also helping her to sleep soundly during the night and fall *back* to sleep after getting up with the baby. The higher quality of sleep combined with heightened energy and mental focus during the day helped Kristen to regain her sense of relaxation and emotional balance.

In addition to these mental aspects of cortisol control, the exercise, nutrition, and supplements in Kristen's personalized SENSE plan helped her modulate her blood-sugar levels, control her appetite, accelerate her fat metabolism, and lose the weight she had gained during pregnancy. In short, SENSE provided a simple and easy-to-follow framework for Kristen to use in getting her life back under control—and back to the place where she felt it should be.

NUTRITION

What is the first thing many of us do when the stress starts to build up? We pile up our plates—and we usually do it with junk food. Nothing stimulates our cravings for sugar, salt, and fat like a stressful event, but attempting to "eat your way out" is *not* the right approach. An entire book could be devoted to helping a person craft his or her own antistress diet (and many have been; see the Resources section for some recommended reading), but it's possible to get the most dramatic benefits from making a few small changes.

First, eat breakfast! Remember Mom telling you how breakfast was the most important meal of the day? Well, she was right—but not all breakfasts are created equal. Breakfast, like all your meals and snacks throughout the day, should be a blend of carbohydrates and protein, with a little bit of fat thrown in. A good rule of thumb is to compose each meal or snack by "fists." Here's how it works: Each meal (breakfast, lunch, and dinner) is made up of one fist-sized helping of carbohydrates (pasta, bread, cereal), one fist-sized helping of protein (eggs, meat, poultry, fish, tofu), and another fist or two of fruits and vegetables (an apple, a banana, a side salad). Each snack (one each between breakfast and lunch, between lunch and dinner, and between dinner and bedtime) should be built the same way, but the total size of a snack should really be no larger than one fist.

Using this simple "fist" method does a few important things for your diet. Eating this way helps to control blood-sugar levels, regulate appetite, and maintain a high resting metabolic rate throughout the day. Eating this way also forces you to consume more fruits and vegetables, something the National Cancer Institute has been telling us to do for a long time (they recommend a minimum of five daily servings of fruits and vegetables). Fruits and veggies are also rich in the vitamins and minerals our bodies need at higher levels during stressful times.

Over the years that we have conducted the SENSE program, we have refined this general "fist" guideline into a more precise framework for eating that we call the Helping Hand approach. It still uses your hands as a portion-control device (helping you gauge the *quantity* that you eat), but it also places some emphasis on the *quality* of the foods in your diet (for optimal metabolism).

Eating for Quality **and** Quantity

Hundreds of clinical studies show that if you eat in "X" manner, you'll lose weight—but that weight often comes right back, and it comes back more often than it stays off. There are also millions of personal testimonials to support the weight-loss benefits of the various miracle diets, no matter how bizarre they may seem (including all manner of patches, potions, and pills). Without too much effort, it is easy to find diets that promise weight loss by restricting a person's intake of a particular food (such as those "bad" carbohydrates), and others that restrict intake of all foods except those on a certain "approved food list" (which invariably tends to be an arbitrary list with little basis in credible scientific evidence).

All Diets Work—for a While

Let's emphasize one very important fact right here at the start: Virtually *any* diet program will help you lose weight. Whether we're talking about Atkins, Protein Power, Zone, Ornish, Pritikin, South Beach, Paleo, or any of the myriad other choices out there, they will *all* help you lose weight. Why? Because they all restrict total energy intake to about fifteen hundred calories per day. Do that (restrict calories) on a consistent basis for any length of time (more than a few days), and the vast majority of Americans (or non-Americans eating a "modern American diet") will shed pounds with very little effort.

It's when you get to those final ten or twenty pounds of desired weight loss that most diets become less effective—and in some cases these diets actually become counterproductive to your weight-loss efforts. Why? Because most of them target only a single aspect of your metabolism to help you lose weight. And while controlling one aspect of metabolism may be sufficient during the early (easy) stages of weight loss, it becomes woefully inadequate in the later (more difficult) stages—when your weight loss begins to plateau, eventually stops, and often starts to reverse toward weight regain.

Those "Last Twenty Pounds"

It goes without saying that the later stages (those last few pounds) are the hardest stages of weight loss—and the ones that cause us the most physical difficulty and mental anguish. Because weight loss gets harder and harder to achieve as we move closer and closer to our goal weight, we need to *simultaneously target multiple metabolic systems* to arrive at our ultimate goal (recall the 3S approach outlined earlier in this chapter). For the vast majority of us, the metabolic systems that are most closely associated with those last ten to twenty pounds involve cortisol (the primary catabolic stress hormone), testosterone (the primary anabolic hormone), and HSD (the cortisol amplifier in fat cells that leads to more fat storage).

Eating SENSE-ibly

The SENSE approach to eating is not about following a strict meal-planning regimen, nor is it about restricting any foods or categories of foods. In fact, it's not much of a "diet" at all. Most of the people who have tried it can confirm that they often eat *more* food while following it—and they still lose weight. SENSE teaches you how to balance your intake of carbohydrates, protein, fat, and fiber in a way that considers both the quantity of food (as all weight-loss diets must do) and, even more importantly, the quality of those foods. Specifically, *quality* refers to what you eat, and *quantity* refers to how much you eat. Don't worry about trying to stick to eating only certain items from a long list of "approved" foods (because all foods are fair game) or avoiding other foods on some "banned" list (because no foods are prohibited).

Quality: What to Eat

Step 1—Consider Carbohydrates
General rule: Foods that are more "whole" (in their natural, unprocessed state) are preferred choices.
Carbohydrates, in and of themselves, are not "bad," but the form of carbohydrate that you choose will determine your body's metabolic response and your likelihood of storing that food as fat. Here are some examples of this principle in action:

- A whole apple is less processed than applesauce, which is less processed than apple juice—so the apple is the best choice, the applesauce is moderate, and the apple juice is least preferred.

- All whole fruits and vegetables are a good choice, and thus can be used to "balance" a food that is less preferred (such as a juicy Italian sausage sandwich at the company picnic—see below).

- Whole-grain forms of high-carbohydrate foods are always preferred over forms that use highly refined grains. When choosing breads, pastas, and crackers, always look at the label for "whole-grain flour" or "whole-wheat flour" and choose these products instead of ones that simply state "wheat flour," which indicates a more highly refined flour rather than a whole-grain flour.

- When you can't examine a label (such as when eating out), choose grain products that are thicker, chewier, and heartier—such as "peasant breads," with added seeds, nuts, and fruits—rather than "fluffier" and "softer" breads, which indicate highly refined grains.

- Choosing whole, unrefined fruits, vegetables, and grains over processed versions of these foods will naturally boost your fiber intake, another important part of the SENSE approach to eating (see Step 4, below).

Step 2—Provide Protein
General rule: Any form of lean protein can be used to "complete" a refined carbohydrate.

- Protein and carbs are the "yin and yang" of nutrition: They have to be consumed together for proper dietary balance (which falls apart when either one is excluded or inappropriately restricted).

- Leaner sources of protein are always a better choice than fattier cuts (choose 97 percent lean ground beef instead of 85 percent lean).

- A bagel for breakfast is not necessarily a "bad" carbohydrate, but it is not the best choice (especially if it's made from refined, white flour instead of whole-wheat flour). Your bagel can be made "better" from a metabolic standpoint by adding some protein—perhaps in the form of smoked salmon or a scrambled egg. The combination of virtually any protein with a refined-carb food balances the meal into one with a better overall metabolic profile— meaning that your body will handle the calories more appropriately.

- Some foods might masquerade as protein—such as bacon, sausage, hot dogs, kielbasa, cheese, nuts, and peanut butter—but their very high fat content means that we treat them as "added fat" and consider how they affect our overall intake (discussed in Step 3).

Step 3—Finish with Fat
General rule: A small amount of added fat at each meal is a "metabolic regulator."

- A bit of added fat—in the form of a pat of butter, a dash of olive oil, a square of cheese, or a handful of nuts—helps to slow the postmeal rise in cortisol and blood sugar, which in turn helps you control appetite and enhances fat burning throughout the day.

- Your choice of pasta as a side dish (but not as a main meal—see the quantity discussion in the next section) is an "okay" choice, but you can make it a better choice by selecting whole-grain pasta (instead of the typical highly refined forms) and/or by topping it with a delicious olive oil, garlic, and basil sauce. Even better, mix some fresh vegetables into the sauce to further boost the nutritional content of the entire meal.

- Your child's lunch of white bread with grape jelly is a metabolic disaster (you might as well inject sugar straight into her veins and fat into her adipose tissue), but you can boost the nutritional content and her body's ability to metabolize her sandwich by adding a bit of peanut butter, insisting that she wash it down with a glass of 1 percent milk, and switching to whole-wheat bread (a tough switch with many kids, but well worth the try).

Step 4—Fill Up with Fiber
General rule: Choosing "whole" forms of grains, fruits, and vegetables (as recommended in Step 1) will automatically satisfy your fiber needs.
Like fat, fiber helps to slow the absorption of sugar from the digestive tract into the bloodstream. In this way, fiber can also be considered a "metabolic regulator" to help balance cortisol and blood-sugar levels at each meal or snack. The fiber content of whole foods also provides a great deal of "satiety"—that is, foods high in fiber make us feel fuller for longer, so we are less likely to feel hungry and to seek out snacks.

Quantity: How Much to Eat—
The "Helping Hand" Approach to Eating

At the same time that you are evaluating the quality aspects of your food choices, you should also be considering the second part of the nutrition equation: quantity (otherwise known as "portion control"). When we talk about food selection for weight control, we know without a doubt that size matters! Luckily, Mother Nature was looking out for your waistline when she equipped you with a handy pair of built-in portion-control devices. You probably know them as your hands. This fortunate turn of events means that we have no excuse to overeat, because we can use our hands to guide us in the quantity part of the SENSE program. It works like this:

Carbohydrates

General rule: Whenever possible, select "whole" and "least processed" carbohydrate sources—but only eat a certain quantity of them.

Fruits and vegetables (except potatoes, which count as concentrated carbs)—Choose a quantity of fruits and vegetables that roughly matches the size of your open hand. Select brightly colored fruits and vegetables for the highest levels of disease-fighting carotenoids (orange, red, yellow) and flavonoids (green, blue, and purple).

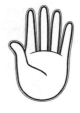

Starches, i.e., bread, cereal, pasta, and other concentrated carb sources (including potatoes and French fries)—Choose a quantity that is no larger than your tightly closed fist (a small side dish of pasta, potato salad, a dinner roll, etc.).

Protein

General rule: Whenever possible, avoid consuming any carbohydrates (whether whole-grain or refined) without added protein and fat.

Lean proteins such as eggs, low-fat yogurt, low-fat milk, lean ground beef, steak (with visible fat trimmed), fish (any), chicken, pork chops, etc.—Choose an amount that approximately matches the size of the palm of your hand. (Note that I said *palm*. I am not referring to your entire open hand.)

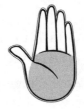

Keep in mind that this portion is likely to be only about half the size of the standard portions served in many American restaurants—so be prepared to eat half and bring the other half home as leftovers.

Fat

General rule: Whenever possible, avoid consuming carbohydrates (whether whole-grain or refined) without added protein and fat.

Any source of fat will do. This means that butter, olive oil, flaxseed oil, canola oil, cheese, and nuts are fine. Make an okay sign with your thumb and index finger, and choose an amount of fat about the size of the circle made by your index finger/thumb.

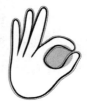

The Helping Hand approach to eating considers both the quality and the quantity of every meal and snack—and the best part is that it requires *zero* counting of calories, fat grams, or carb grams. Why? Because the calorie control is already built in, based on the size of your hands (Mother Nature's automatic portion control). So a person with average-sized hands (and likely an average-sized body and metabolism) will consume about 500 calories from each meal planned using the balance-factor hand approach. Smaller individuals (with smaller hands and lower metabolic rates) will eat slightly smaller meals, amounting to approximately 400 calories each, while larger people (with larger hands and higher metabolic rates) will eat slightly larger meals, amounting to closer to 600 calories each. Eat this way at breakfast, lunch, and dinner and you'll consume about 1,200 to 1,800 calories each day—precisely the same range of calories associated with the very best long-term weight-loss success.

Timing: When to Eat

The last aspect of eating "SENSE-ibly" that we need to discuss is timing, or when to eat—and the SENSE approach represents a subtle but important departure from many popular diets. Like many existing programs, SENSE encourages you to eat several small meals and snacks throughout the day. This approach to eating can do wonders for helping to modulate your blood sugar and cortisol responses to food, thereby helping to control appetite, boost energy levels, and encourage fat burning throughout the day.

SENSE optimizes this approach by spacing three meals and three snacks throughout the day in the following pattern:

7 A.M.: Snack (before leaving for work)

9 A.M.: Breakfast (at work)

Noon: Snack (plus exercise if you can fit it in)

2 P.M.: Lunch (postexercise)

5 P.M.: Snack (before leaving work or on the way home)

7 P.M.: Dinner (with a small cocktail or a small dessert as your optional fourth "snack" of the day)

A "snack" consists of one appropriately sized serving from the fruit/veggie group, plus one appropriately sized serving of fat (for example, an apple and a piece of cheese). A "meal" consists of one appropriately sized serving from each of the carb/starch, protein, and fat groups, plus one or two appropriately sized servings from the fruit/veggie group.

Note: From a weight-loss perspective, a snack can consist of one serving from any of the groups, but from an overall health perspective, it is better if the snack consists of one serving from the fruit/veggie group plus one serving of fat. This combination delivers more fiber and important phytonutrients that are less likely to be found in a protein or starch serving (though whole-grain starches would not be a bad second choice, because they also contain phytonutrients such as lignans).

You'll notice that each snack "lasts" for two hours, until it is time for a meal that "lasts" for three hours. The snacks and meals are spaced out in this manner because I have found this to work best for the majority of the busy professionals who come to me for nutrition consultation and diet design. Not many of us are able to sit down to a relaxing breakfast before heading out the door for work; breakfast is usually something obtained at a drive-through and gulped down on the way to rush-hour traffic. Likewise, most of us aren't able to make it home from work with enough time to watch the evening news, prepare dinner, and enjoy a meal anytime before seven at night. This schedule also works very well for the participants in our research studies of the SENSE Lifestyle Program. It leads many participants to remark that they feel like they are "always" eating and "never" hungry, and yet they still lose fat and inches. In this scenario, your snacks act as "bridges" between meals and as significant controllers of cortisol, blood sugar, and overall metabolic rate. Do not neglect them!

That's it—and it is hard to get any simpler than the Helping Hand approach to eating. At this point, you can see how this method can be easy to follow, practical to use in your everyday life, and effective as a way to control the key aspects of metabolism that are keeping many of us from losing those last ten to twenty pounds.

If there was one thing in the world that caused *Marta* a high level of stress, it was her distress at her inability to lose those "last ten pounds" of body fat from around her hips and buttocks. Marta was a veteran of just about every fad diet in existence, but nothing seemed to work. As a self-described "stress monster," Marta was attracted to the SENSE program because it combined both physical and mental aspects of health. Marta felt that she needed help to balance her eating habits with her exercise regimen (don't we all), but she was intimidated by the "no pain, no gain" mentality that she encountered at her local gym. As someone who was also prone to anxiety attacks, the last thing that Type C Marta needed was a Type A fitness trainer pushing her through an aggressive exercise regimen. Instead, Marta opted for an approach to exercise that helped her to feel more relaxed, less stressed, and more focused.

Marta's approach to the exercise problem was to largely "forget about it" and focus on simply getting in as many miles of walking as possible in a given week. Marta bought a small pedometer to record the number of steps she took each day—and she made it her goal to record as many steps as possible. Taking the "forget about it" approach to exercising, Marta removed a primary source of stress (and excess cortisol) from her life. Marta's newfound cortisol control allowed her body to readjust its metabolic profile, and tighter blood-sugar control, better control over appetite, and accelerated fat metabolism were the primary outcomes that inched Marta toward her ultimate goal of saying good-bye to those "last ten pounds" for good.

Instead of focusing on the exercise portion of the SENSE program, Marta chose to focus her efforts on the nutrition (N), supplement (S), and evaluation (E) aspects of the plan. In terms of nutrition, Marta went on an aggressive regimen of meal replacements (plus a daily multivitamin/multimineral supplement). Shakes and bars replaced breakfast, lunch, and two snacks for four weeks; a healthy dinner was the only "real" meal that Marta prepared for the entire month. Following that initial four-week period, Marta reevaluated her efforts and her goals. She had lost a little more than five pounds of body weight—and a body-fat analysis indicated that 80 percent of her weight loss up to that point was from fat—so Marta was about halfway to her goal and certainly on the right track.

The only complaint she noted during her first four weeks was a craving for sweets in the late afternoon and in the evening before bed, so she felt that perhaps she needed to increase her total calorie consumption by just a bit in the next phase (six weeks). This slight increase in calorie consumption came from incorporating more "real" foods into her diet. Dinner remained the same balanced meal of one fist-sized piece of protein (such as salmon), one fist-sized serving of carbohydrates (such as rice), and two fist-sized servings of salad or steamed vegetables. But Marta now followed the same balancing guidelines (while cutting the fist-sized portions in half) when she made her lunchtime sandwich (whole-grain roll, turkey, lettuce, tomato, sprouts, and low-fat mayo).

During this six-week period, Marta noted that her cravings for sweets had vanished. But even more important was her continued weight loss, which topped out at twelve pounds lost (90 percent of it from body fat) in just ten weeks. Marta had exceeded her weight-loss goals—an objective she had failed to achieve on numerous occasions in the past—and the primary difference between then and now was the more relaxed and balanced approach she'd followed.

Now it was time for another evaluation period. This time Marta needed to decide whether to try to continue with additional weight loss or simply attempt to maintain what she had already accomplished. Knowing that weight *maintenance* can be much more difficult for many people than the initial weight *loss,* Marta was feeling a bit apprehensive about the possibility that she might gain back all of her lost weight. As a way to counteract her growing anxiety (which could increase her cortisol levels and set the stage for weight regain), she continued with a daily nutrition program that looked like this:

Breakfast: Meal-replacement shake plus multivitamin/ mineral supplement (250 calories)

Morning snack: Energy bar (160 calories)

Lunch: Turkey sandwich (380 calories)

Afternoon snack: Handful of nuts and glass of water (180 calories)

Dinner: Grilled chicken with steamed rice and vegetables (520 calories)

Evening snack: Chocolate milk with piece of fruit (240 calories)

TOTAL CALORIES: 1,730

In addition to her balanced nutrition regimen, Marta added a twice-daily supplement of magnolia bark extract to her morning and evening snacks. The mild antianxiety effects of magnolia helped Marta to stay focused and remain calm about her switch to a slightly higher-calorie weight-maintenance regimen, making it so she didn't get stressed out and her cortisol levels stayed in their normal ranges.

To many of her friends, Marta is now one of those "lucky" people who is able to "effortlessly" maintain her new, slimmer figure without much attention to diet or exercise. More than once she has been told that she must have "good genes" to be able to eat the way she does (to some, it looks as if she eats all the time), take a laissez-faire attitude toward high-intensity exercise, and generally seem unconcerned and relaxed about the whole public furor over body weight.

Sample Menu Plan for Meals and Snacks

Remember that we need to space our meals and snacks throughout the day to help regulate cortisol metabolism. Follow the general plan outlined in the table below and in the "Further Guidelines" section, but substitute foods that you prefer (e.g., turkey for roast beef on your sandwich, or sushi instead of salmon at dinner), or foods that you have ready access to (such as when eating away from home).

Sample Menu Plan for Meals and Snacks

Time	Meal	Fruit/Veggie	Starch	Protein	Fat
7 A.M.	Snack	Banana	N/A	N/A	Peanut butter
9 A.M.	Breakfast	Grapefruit (+2 teaspoons of added sugar, optional)	Shredded wheat cereal	1% milk	Coffee with half & half
Noon	Snack	Apple	N/A	N/A	Block of cheese
2 P.M.	Lunch	3 tomato slices, 1 leaf Romaine lettuce, 1 pear	2 slices whole-wheat bread	Lean roast beef	Swiss cheese and mustard to taste
5 P.M.	Snack	Baby carrots	N/A	N/A	Salad dressing
7 P.M.	Dinner	½ cup of green beans and ½ cup of carrots seasoned with olive oil and garlic	1 whole-wheat dinner roll	Salmon fillet	Olive oil with garlic (for the roll and fish)
9 P.M.	Dessert (see **Further Guidelines** on the next page)	Air-popped popcorn	N/A	N/A	Melted butter

Further Guidelines

Number of portions: A *snack* consists of **one** appropriately sized serving from the fruit/veggie group, plus **one** appropriately sized serving of fat. A *meal* consists of **one** appropriately sized serving from **each** of the starch, protein, and fat groups, plus **one or two** appropriately sized servings from the fruit/veggie group.

Fluids: An eight-ounce glass of water is suggested at each meal and snack. (Eight fluid ounces = one cup.)

Sleep prescription: 10:30 P.M. to 6:00 A.M.—i.e., get at least 7.5 hours nightly for optimal cortisol control.

Exercise prescription: Thirty to sixty minutes of activity, three to five times per week, for optimal control of cortisol, testosterone, and growth hormone.

Fruit/veggie guideline: Remember, "Choose it if it's bright, and forget it if it's white." This will guide you toward brightly colored choices that are better sources of antioxidants and essential phytonutrients.

Starch (concentrated carbohydrate) guideline: Select minimally processed, dark, thick, coarse, and chewy forms of grains over their highly refined counterparts (white, light, smooth, puffed, and fluffy).

Protein guideline: Choose lean cuts of meat, poultry, pork, and fish.

Fat guideline: Don't skip fat to save a few calories; instead, add it to meals and snacks as a metabolic regulator. Avoid trans-fats in the form of hydrogenated oils in processed foods.

Dessert guideline (bonus!): If you have exercised for thirty to sixty minutes on a particular day, then as your optional fourth snack of the day, add either a cocktail or a glass of wine or beer with dinner, or a fist-sized dessert after dinner. If you have not exercised, then skip the alcohol and end dinner with a piece of fresh fruit instead.

Following the Helping Hand approach helps you balance the *quality* of your food choices with the *quantity* of those choices, so you regulate calories to approximately 1,500 per day (typical range = 1,200–1,800 calories), which are obtained from a balanced intake of about 55 percent carbohydrates, 20 percent protein, and 25 percent fat. Remember that these are exactly the levels associated with the most dramatic weight loss and longest-lasting weight maintenance in the largest research studies.

SUPPLEMENTATION

Although this book focuses a great deal on controlling the stress response and cortisol levels using dietary supplements, it is important to (re)emphasize that supplements fall *fourth* in the whole scheme of things—behind stress management, regular exercise, and optimal nutrition. From a practical point of view, however, many of us simply do not have the ability, time, or inclination to live the "perfect" antistress lifestyle—and in these situations, supplements play a more prominent role.

So, *after* doing what you can do in terms of stress avoidance/management, getting adequate amounts of sleep and exercise, and eating a balanced diet, *then* turn your attention to using dietary supplements to help control cortisol. When you begin to focus on the supplement side of things, it makes sense to approach them step-by-step, as follows:

Step 1

Avoid excessive doses of supplements that can increase cortisol levels. These tend to be ingredients that fall into the category of herbal stimulants, and they are often found in weight-loss and appetite-suppressant products. These supplements, *when used at appropriate doses*, certainly appear to offer a small benefit for promoting weight loss by controlling appetite, increasing energy levels, and boosting thermogenesis (calorie burning). When used in excessive doses or for extended periods of time, however, they will increase cortisol levels, disrupt blood-sugar levels, increase appetite, and sabotage efforts at long-term weight control.

Step 2

Take a comprehensive multivitamin/multimineral supplement. In particular, the supplement you choose should provide adequate amounts of the most important antistress nutrients that are needed at increased levels during periods of high stress: vitamin C, magnesium, calcium, and the B-complex vitamins. Your multivitamin/ multimineral supplement will provide the foundation of your cortisol-control supplement regimen, so the more comprehensive it is, providing the full range of essential nutrients, the better.

Step 3

Focus on targeted cortisol-modulating supplements. This is where you'll be able to make the most dramatic gains toward maintaining healthy cortisol levels using supplements. Of the many supplements that may play a role in modulating the stress response and controlling cortisol levels, the most direct and promising benefits are likely to come from eurycoma, PMFs, magnolia bark, and theanine.

This is as far as most people will need to go in terms of using supplements to help control cortisol levels. When these are used in the context of the entire SENSE program, they help keep cortisol levels in an optimal range so that you reap the long-term health benefits. During times of particularly high stress, however, additional supplements can be used to provide a temporary "control point" designed to rebalance the stress response. The supplements addressed in Chapter 8 include a variety of adaptogens, as well as relaxation and calming supplements that can help reinforce your body against heightened stress, depression, anxiety, and insomnia on a short-term basis.

> After learning about the detrimental health effects of chronically elevated cortisol, *Mario* joked that cortisol was his middle name—but he was serious about his desire to get his cortisol

levels under control. As a long-haul truck driver, Mario experienced the quadruple threat of high stress (time pressure to deliver his loads on time), inadequate exercise, poor nutrition, and irregular sleep patterns. As a textbook case for elevated cortisol levels, Mario was certainly about as extreme as they come.

On the stress-management end of things, Mario had a heck of a long way to go. As an extreme Type C personality, his highest cortisol exposure generally occurred during traffic jams, when he sat and virtually boiled in his own stress hormones. Mario's chief problem with traffic was that it kept him from meeting his tight schedule—and consequently he felt helpless and stressed whenever the traffic slowed to a crawl. After he tried a number of stress-management approaches (breathing exercises, positive imagery, music, books on tape, and others), the solution that finally worked for Mario was to talk to his family and friends on his cell phone. As it turns out, part of the reason why traffic caused Mario to experience such high stress was because he felt that it was another obstacle keeping him from spending time with his loved ones (and it was an obstacle that he could do little to influence). As a result, when the traffic slowed, Mario's stress increased—and so did his cortisol, his cholesterol, his appetite, and his waistline. The cell phone, along with unlimited long-distance minutes and a hands-free attachment to allow him to keep both hands on the wheel, allowed Mario to stay in touch with his wife, kids, and friends—and became a significant de-stressing mechanism whenever he felt that he might be delayed. Even a conversation lasting a few minutes was enough for Mario and his family to stay mentally and emotionally connected during his frequent extended trips.

Now that the primary source of Mario's stress was identified and partially controlled, our attention turned to giving him a "supercharge" in terms of targeted cortisol control. Because his need to stay alert during the day was literally a matter of life and death (you don't want a drowsy driver behind the wheel of an eighteen-wheeler traveling at seventy miles per hour), some of the traditional antistress supplements (kava, valerian, melatonin) were ruled out because of their sedating effects. Instead,

Mario started using theanine in the evening (200 mg taken as soon as he pulled his truck over for the night) as a way to relax him and help him fall asleep faster and stay asleep through the night. A significant side benefit of theanine was that he felt no "morning after" effects such as sluggishness or sleepiness, so he woke up refreshed and ready to face the long day ahead. Besides Mario's reports that he was feeling better (with more energy and clearer thinking), the increase in the quantity and quality of his sleep helped his body to better regulate its own cortisol levels (they slowly fell during the evening hours).

The second phase of supplementation for Mario was his incorporation of a daily multivitamin/multimineral along with a phosphatidylserine (PS) supplement in the morning and a beta-sitosterol (BS) supplement (also known as *phytosterols*) in the evening. The multi provided a general antistress foundation on which the PS and BS could begin to control cortisol levels. The morning dosing of PS took advantage of its dual effects in controlling cortisol and boosting brainpower and concentration (nice side effects for a truck driver in an unfamiliar city). The evening dosing of BS produced the dual effects of controlling cortisol and reducing cholesterol levels (Mario's largest and fattiest meal of the day was almost always dinner, which he would eat at a roadside diner). The cholesterol-lowering effect of BS occurs at a much higher level (about 3 grams per day) than the cortisol-controlling effects (60–120 mg per day), but BS is perfectly safe, and four large capsules at dinner were not much of an inconvenience to Mario—especially given the fact that BS can block a large amount of cholesterol from being absorbed.

Mario enjoyed success in controlling his primary sources of cortisol overexposure (stressing out about traffic delays and getting inadequate sleep), but what about his diet and exercise patterns? It might surprise you that Mario's strategy in these areas was to do very little at all. We learned early on that a strict diet and exercise regimen was not only unrealistic for Mario's work and travel schedule, but it would also have represented an additional source of daily stress for him to deal with. Instead, the exercise piece of the puzzle was limited to walking on as many days of the week as possible when he was at home with his family (walks around the neighborhood became a sort of family event). The nutrition part of SENSE was also quite limited in its scope; it centered on counteracting Mario's tendency to snack on convenience foods in the cab of his truck. To this end, Mario agreed to focus his snacking on balanced foods—so donuts were replaced by whole-grain bagels with peanut butter, cupcakes were replaced by energy bars containing both carbohydrates and protein, and potato chips were replaced by a handful of mixed nuts.

After just a few days on the SENSE program, Mario noticed an immediate change in how he felt; the key benefits were sounder sleep, more energy, and a clearer mind. Within two weeks, Mario's appetite and eating habits came back into balance and he was able to start focusing on getting his body weight under control. Even without a "perfect" diet and exercise regimen, the fact that Mario had regained control over his body's stress response and cortisol levels made it possible for him to lose five inches off his waistline in a little less than six months. Mario still has a long way to go to get down to his ideal body weight, but with his cortisol-control issues out of the way, he is headed in the right direction.

EVALUATION

It is important to keep in mind that neither a person's stress levels nor the body's response to stress is a constant. Instead, there will be periods in each of our lives when we experience more stress or less stress—just as there will be times when we feel as if we can withstand stress better than other times. Accordingly, the last step in the SENSE program, evaluation, reminds us that we need to alter our exercise patterns, nutrient intake, and supplementation regimen according to our exposure to stress. For example, regular exercise and a balanced diet are always going to be important, but they become even more so during stressful times. Skipping breakfast during a period of low stress isn't ideal, but it isn't going to kill you. Skip that balanced breakfast during a high-stress period, however, and you're setting yourself up for poor blood-sugar control, surges in appetite, and feelings of fatigue—each of which will be even more pronounced because of your high-stress profile.

So how do you evaluate your current stress profile? Take the Type C Self-Test included in the Introduction to get a good baseline gauge of your stress exposure and your cortisol levels—and then take it again every three months to reevaluate where you stand. Are you experiencing higher than normal stress levels? If so, then your cortisol levels are likely to be elevated, and you need to be especially careful about following each step of the SENSE program to keep your cortisol levels within a healthy range. Alternatively, are you enjoying an interlude that's relatively stress-free and tranquil? If this is the case, then perhaps you can be less vigilant about every aspect of SENSE, and relax and take pleasure in the welcome fruits of the healthy lifestyle you've created by following the sound stress-management, sleep, exercise, nutritional, and supplementation habits promoted by the SENSE plan. And once you've reached this point, having created healthy new habits and having witnessed how they've benefited you, you'll be more motivated than ever to maintain them as part of your daily life.

CONCLUDING WORDS

I hope this book has made clear that cortisol is a necessary hormone, but also that cortisol levels elevated too high for too long will leave you feeling bad and looking bad, and put you on the fast track toward a long list of chronic diseases. These conditions run the gamut from simple feelings of fatigue and forgetfulness to more serious debilitations such as obesity, diabetes, cancer, cardiovascular disease, and depression.

The good news, however, is that following the SENSE Lifestyle Program outlined in this book can help you control your body's response to your many daily stressors, so that cortisol levels are maintained in a healthier range. Using SENSE will help you lose weight, maintain muscle mass, boost energy levels, improve mood, reduce the frequency of illness, increase brainpower, and enhance your sex drive.

As the scientific and medical research linking cortisol and disease continues to advance, additional wisdom will undoubtedly be discovered that we can all incorporate into our personal SENSE programs. I wish you the best in doing so, and in maintaining healthy cortisol levels and optimizing your long-term health.

. . . .
. .
. .
. .

Putting the SENSE Lifestyle Program to the Test

How do I know that the SENSE Lifestyle Program will work for you? Because it has been studied, and it has been *proven* to work in groups of the toughest cases we could find. These tough cases were people who had tried every popular diet and exercise craze and yet still found themselves with extra weight to lose. They were people who had counted the calories, and the fat grams, and the carb grams—but the weight remained. They were people who had been exercising religiously all along, some of them even partnering with a personal trainer in an effort to "force" those pounds away with extremes of exercise—but again, to no avail. The pounds stayed put. Not until these people followed the SENSE program did they find the solution—and the success—they had been looking for.

As a scientist, I find that theories and ideas are nice, but cold hard evidence is where the rubber meets the road. In the words of many of my colleagues, I want to "see the data" about a particular program before I will believe it works. Based on the data, other professionals can recommend a given program with a certain degree of confidence that it will actually work for their clients and patients. So over the last handful of years I have felt very strongly about continuing to put the SENSE Lifestyle Program to the test to see if these ideas would really stand up to the harsh reality of losing weight in the real world. It all makes "sense" on paper from a biochemical and physiological perspective, but there have been lots of great ideas on paper that never made a lick of difference to anyone in the real world.

With the general plan for SENSE developed, and with the invaluable assistance of AnneMarie Christopulos and Wayne Larsen at the Treehouse Athletic Club in Draper, Utah, we have followed group after group of participants (more than a thousand satisfied customers at last count) over the last five years. SENSE has been offered in six-week, eight-week, and twelve-week versions—and we always set out to recruit as many "hard cases" as we can find. By "hard cases," I mean people who in the past had tried and tried and tried to lose weight with other programs and who just could not seem to succeed. Why would we recruit the toughest cases and seemingly set ourselves up for failure? Simply because based on my experience conducting weight-loss trials over the past decade or so, it is generally easy to recruit a group of extremely overweight subjects and get them to lose large amounts of weight in a short period of time; almost any simplified program of diet or exercise will do it. With SENSE, I'm trying to help the millions of Americans who struggle day in and day out with that ten or twenty or thirty pounds of weight that simply won't respond to simplified diets and exercise regimens. It's these folks who need help cracking their weight-loss code—and SENSE has been repeatedly put to the test to help them.

As part of following the SENSE program, our participants would meet periodically to talk about how cortisol, testosterone, diet, exercise, and supplements could have an impact on mood, energy, appetite, and weight-loss success. We measured body weight, body fat, waist circumference, cortisol and testosterone levels, cholesterol values, and stress/anxiety levels.

The results were nothing short of dramatic. Not only did virtually every person in the program lose body weight, body fat, and inches around their midsection, but the majority of people also reported increased feelings of energy, reduced stress/anxiety, control of appetite and cravings, and no feelings of deprivation. The most common comment about SENSE (and it's one we hear a lot) is that nobody feels like they are on a "diet," and yet they continue to lose weight, fat, and inches. Plus, they feel great doing it.

Of particular interest with SENSE is the fact that taking a dietary supplement for controlling stress, cortisol, testosterone, and HSD (in addition to following the diet and exercise prescriptions) seemed to help participants to lose more weight/fat and more inches from their waist compared to when they had tried their own versions of diet and exercise alone. In no way does this mean that the supplement was a substitute for diet and exercise, but it suggests strongly that by adding the supplement to their diet and exercise regimen, they were able to reap some additional metabolic control and thus enjoy a greater degree of weight loss. In many ways, the results make perfect "sense," because taking a supplement means that you have additional factors driving you toward weight loss (compared to relying on diet and exercise alone). The bottom-line effects of SENSE show us that it helps people lose more of those stubborn "last few pounds"—even if these people have been struggling with those pounds for a long time.

RESULTS

The fact that a new "popular" diet (that is, one written for the real world and for real people) has been studied so extensively for several years comes as quite a surprise to most of my colleagues. The typical course of events is for some diet "guru" to write a book with lots of miraculous claims (lose weight and eat all you want!), for the author and publisher to hook up with a marketing outfit, and for the book to ride the top of the best-seller charts until people figure out that it doesn't really work as promised. In the case of SENSE, I was prepared to put my money where my mouth was so that when my colleagues said, "Show me the data," I could do just that.

When we look across the last five years of conducting the SENSE program on approximately one thousand subjects, we generally find the following results:

- Individuals lose about one-half to one pound of *fat* each week. I say "fat" instead of just "weight" because it's important to know that our participants are losing the fat and keeping the muscle—meaning they are thinner and healthier, but they maintain their metabolic rate, which helps them keep the weight off.

- Cortisol level drops and testosterone level rises, resulting in a rebalancing of the cortisol-to-testosterone ratio toward one that favors fat loss and muscle maintenance. Our SENSE participants generally see a change in this C:T ratio of 15–20 percent, and it is one of the major biochemical effects that makes them feel so good, experiencing elevated mood, abundant energy, and clear thinking.

- Metabolic rate stays exactly the same, meaning that SENSE prevents the drop in metabolism that you would expect with a standard weight-loss diet. This happens because the participant's hormones are balanced and his/her muscle mass is preserved, whereas on many other diets, hormones become disrupted and the person loses muscle.

- Cholesterol (both total cholesterol and "bad," or LDL, cholesterol) falls by about 20 percent. This is partly due to better eating, partly due to hormone maintenance, and partly due to a gradual loss of body fat.

- Mood and energy levels increase and depression and tension levels decrease, often by an astonishing amount (15–50 percent), due to the maintenance of hormone profiles and the fact that participants are losing fat without depriving themselves.

Perhaps the most striking statistic from our studies of SENSE—even more exciting than the fat loss, the maintenance of hormones and metabolism, or even the significant drop in cholesterol levels—is the extremely high compliance rate (indicating how many people actually finish SENSE and lose weight). Our compliance rate of

91 percent is higher than any other program I have ever encountered. Most of the popular "diet book" programs, from Atkins to South Beach to Zone, and even Weight Watchers, have compliance rates of around 50 percent.

The data from our various offerings of SENSE have been presented at some of the top nutrition-science conferences in the world, including the International Congress on Nutrition and Fitness, the American College of Nutrition, Experimental Biology, the American College of Sports Medicine, the International Society for Sports Nutrition, and the North American Society for the Study of Obesity. Attendees at these research conferences generally find that the most interesting feature of the SENSE Lifestyle Program is not any single aspect of the program, but rather that the synergy between the component parts is so effective when melded into a single approach. For example, we've known for years that regular exercise and a balanced diet are the foundation of a healthy weight-management program, but what SENSE shows is that by building on the diet/exercise foundation with attention to balanced metabolism (of cortisol, testosterone, HSD, and the rest), the "standard" weight-loss results of diet plus exercise can be optimized, much to the delight of SENSE adherents.

References

Chapters 1–3 and 6–7:
Stress, Cortisol Metabolism, and Disease

Abelson, J. L., and G. C. Curtis. "Hypothalamic-Pituitary-Adrenal Axis Activity in Panic Disorder: 24-Hour Secretion of Corticotropin and Cortisol." *Archives of General Psychiatry*, April 1996, 53(4): 323–31.

Al'Alabsi, M., and D. K. Arnett. "Adrenocortical Responses to Psychological Stress and Risk for Hypertension." *Biomedical Pharmacotherapy*, June 2000, 54(5): 234–44.

Andrew, R., D. I. Phillips, and B. R. Walker. "Obesity and Gender Influences on Cortisol Secretion and Metabolism in Man." *Journal of Clinical Endocrinology and Metabolism*, May 1998, 83(5): 1806–9.

Balestreri, R., G. E. Jacopino, E. Foppiani, and N. Elicio. "Aspects of Cortisol Metabolism in Obesity." *Archives of the Maragliano Pathology Clinic*, July–August 1968, 24(4): 431–41.

Balldin, J., K. Blennow, G. Brane, C. G. Gottfries, I. Karlsson, B. Regland, and A. Wallin. "Relationship Between Mental Impairment and HPA Axis Activity in Dementia Disorders." *Dementia*, September–October 1994, 5(5): 252–56.

Biller, B. M., H. J. Federoff, J. I. Koenig, and A. Klibanski. "Abnormal Cortisol Secretion and Responses to Corticotropin-Releasing Hormone in Women with Hypothalamic Amenorrhea." *Journal of Clinical Endocrinology and Metabolism*, February 1990, 70(2): 311–17.

Bjorntorp, P., and R. Rosmond. "Hypothalamic Origin of the Metabolic Syndrome X." *Annual of the New York Academy of Science*, 18 November 1999, 892: 297–307.

Bjorntorp, P., and R. Rosmond. "The Metabolic Syndrome: A Neuroendocrine Disorder?" *British Journal of Nutrition*, March 2000, 83(suppl. 1): S49–57.

Bjorntorp, P., and R. Rosmond. "Obesity and Cortisol." *Nutrition*, October 2000, 16(10): 924–36.

Brillon, D. J., B. Zheng, R. G. Campbell, and D. E. Matthews. "Effect of Cortisol on Energy Expenditure and Amino Acid Metabolism in Humans." *American Journal of Physiology*, March 1995, 268(3 Pt 1):E501–13.

Brindley, D. N. "Neuroendocrine Regulation and Obesity." *International Journal of Obesity and Related Metabolic Disorders*, December 1992, 16(suppl. 3): S73–9.

Catley, D., A. T. Kaell, C. Kirschbaum, and A. A. Stone. "A Naturalistic Evaluation of Cortisol Secretion in Persons with Fibromyalgia and Rheumatoid Arthritis." *Arthritis Care Resources*, February 2000, 13(1): 51–61.

Cauffield, J. S., and H. J. Forbes. "Dietary Supplements Used in the Treatment of Depression, Anxiety, and Sleep Disorders." *Lippincotts Primary Care Practitioner*, May–June 1999, 3(3): 290–304.

Chalew, S., H. Nagel, and S. Shore. "The Hypothalamic-Pituitary-Adrenal Axis in Obesity." *Obesity Resources*, July 1995, 3(4): 371–82.

Chrousos, G. P. "The Role of Stress and the Hypothalamic-Pituitary-Adrenal Axis in the Pathogenesis of the Metabolic Syndrome: Neuro-Endocrine and Target Tissue-Related Causes." *International Journal of Obesity and Related Metabolic Disorders*, June 2000, 24(suppl. 2): S50–55.

Dennison, E., P. Hindmarsh, C. Fall, et al. "Profiles of Endogenous Circulating Cortisol and Bone Mineral Density in Healthy Elderly Men." *Journal of Clinical Endocrinology and Metabolism*, September 1999, 84(9): 3058–63.

Eichner, E. R. "Overtraining: Consequences and Prevention." *Journal of Sports Science*, Summer 1995, 13, spec. no.: S41–48.

Epel, E., R. Lapidus, B. McEwen, and K. Brownell. "Stress May Add Bite to Appetite in Women: A Laboratory Study of Stress-Induced Cortisol and Eating Behavior." *Psychoneuroendocrinology*, January 2001, 26(1):37–49.

Epel, E. E., A. E. Moyer, C. D. Martin, S. Macary, N. Cummings, J. Rodin, and M. Rebuffe-Scrive. "Stress-Induced Cortisol, Mood, and Fat Distribution in Men." *Obesity Resources*, October 2000, 279(4): R1357–64.

Fry, A. C., W. J. Kraemer, and L. T. Ramsey. "Pituitary-Adrenal-Gonadal Responses to High-Intensity Resistance Exercise Overtraining." *Journal of Applied Physiology*, December 1998, 85(6): 2352–59.

Fry, R. W., J. R. Grove, A. R. Morton, P. M. Zeroni, S. Gaudieri, and D. Keast. "Psychological and Immunological Correlates of Acute Over-training." *British Journal of Sports Medicine*, December 1994, 28(4): 241–46.

Holmang, A., and P. Bjorntorp. "The Effects of Cortisol on Insulin Sensitivity in Muscle." *Acta Physiologica Scandinavia*, April 1992, 144(4):425–31.

Jefferies, W. M. "Cortisol and Immunity." *Medical Hypotheses*, March 1991, 34(3): 198–208.

Kelly, G. S. "Nutritional and Botanical Interventions to Assist with the Adaptation to Stress." *Alternative Medicine Review*, August 1999, 4(4): 249–65.

Landsberg, L. "The Sympathoadrenal System, Obesity and Hypertension: An Overview." *Journal of Neuroscience Methods*, September 1990, 34(1–3): 179–86.

Leverenz, J. B., C. W. Wilkinson, M. Wamble, S. Corbin, J. E. Grabber, M. A. Raskind, and E. R. Peskind. "Effect of Chronic High-Dose Exogenous Cortisol on Hippocampal Neuronal Number in Aged Non-human Primates." *Journal of Neuroscience*, 15 March 1999, 19(6): 2356–61.

Lewicka, S., M. Nowicki, and P. Vecsei. "Effect of Sodium Restriction on Urinary Excretion of Cortisol and Its Metabolites in Humans." *Steroids*, July–August 1998, 63(7–8): 401–5.

Ljung, T., G. Holm, P. Friberg, B. Andersson, B. A. Bengtsson, J. Svensson, M. Dallman, B. McEwen, and P. Bjorntorp. "The Activity of the Hypothalamic-Pituitary-Adrenal Axis and the Sympathetic Nervous System in Relation to Waist/Hip Circumference Ratio in Men." *Obesity Resources*, October 2000, 8(7): 487–95.

Lottenberg, S. A., D. Giannella-Neto, H. Derendorf, et al. "Effect of Fat Distribution on the Pharmacokinetics of Cortisol in Obesity." *International Journal of Clinical Pharmacological Therapy*, September 1998, 36(9):501–5.

Marin, P., N. Darin, T. Amemiya, B. Andersson, S. Jern, and P. Bjorntorp. "Cortisol Secretion in Relation to Body-Fat Distribution in Obese Premenopausal Women." *Metabolism*, August 1992, 41(8): 882–86.

Matthews, D. E., and A. Battezzati. "Regulation of Protein Metabolism During Stress." *Current Opinions in General Surgery*, 1993: 72–7.

McLean, J. A., S. I. Barr, and J. C. Prior. "Cognitive Dietary Restraint Is

Associated with Higher Urinary Cortisol Excretion in Healthy Pre-menopausal Women." *American Journal of Clinical Nutrition,* January 2001, 73(1):7–12.

Miller, T. P., J. Taylor, S. Rogerson, M. Mauricio, Q. Kennedy, A. Schatzberg, J. Tinklenberg, and J. Yesavage. "Cognitive and Noncognitive Symptoms in Dementia Patients: Relationship to Cortisol and Dehydroepiandrosterone." *International Psychogeriatrics,* March 1998, 10(1): 85–96.

Mills, F. J. "The Endocrinology of Stress." *Aviation and Space Environmental Medicine,* July 1985, 56(7): 642–50.

Nasman, B., T. Olsson, M. Viitanen, and K. Carlstrom. "A Subtle Disturbance in the Feedback Regulation of the Hypothalamic-Pituitary-Adrenal Axis in the Early Phase of Alzheimer's Disease." *Psychoneuroendocrinology* 1995, 20(2): 211–20.

Piccirillo, G., F. L. Fimognari, V. Infantino, G. Monteleone, G. B. Fimognari, D. Falletti, and V. Marigliano. "High Plasma Concentrations of Cortisol and Thromboxane B2 in Patients with Depression." *American Journal of Medical Science,* March 1994, 307(3): 228–32.

Pirke, K. M., R. J. Tuschl, B. Spyra, et al. "Endocrine Findings in Restrained Eaters." *Physiology and Behavior,* May 1990, 47(5):903–6.

Plotsky, P. M., M. J. Owens, and C. B. Nemeroff. "Psychoneuroendocrinology of Depression: Hypothalamic-Pituitary-Adrenal Axis." *Psychiatric Clinics of North America,* June 1998, 21(2): 293–307.

Raber, J. "Detrimental Effects of Chronic Hypothalamic-Pituitary-Adrenal Axis Activation: From Obesity to Memory Deficits." *Molecular Neurobiology,* August 1998, 18(1): 1–22.

Raff, H., J. L. Raff, E. H. Duthie, et al. "Elevated Salivary Cortisol in the Evening in Healthy Elderly Men and Women: Correlation with Bone Mineral Density." *The Journals of Gerontology. (Series A, Biological Sciences and Medical Sciences),* September 1999, 54(9):M479–83.

Richdale, A. L., and M. R. Prior. "Urinary Cortisol Circadian Rhythm in a Group of High-Functioning Children with Autism." *Journal of Autism and Developmental Disorders,* September 1992, 22(3): 433–47.

Rosmond, R., and P. Bjorntorp. "Blood Pressure in Relation to Obesity, Insulin and the Hypothalamic-Pituitary-Adrenal Axis in Swedish Men." *Journal of Hypertension,* December 1998, 16(12, pt. 1): 1721–26.

Rosmond, R., and P. Bjorntorp. "Occupational Status, Cortisol Secretory Pattern, and Visceral Obesity in Middle-Aged Men." *Obesity Resources,* September 2000, 8(6): 445–50.

Rosmond, R., M. F. Dallman, and P. Bjorntorp. "Stress-Related Cortisol Secretion in Men: Relationships with Abdominal Obesity and Endocrine, Metabolic and Hemodynamic Abnormalities." *Journal of Clinical Endocrinology and Metabolism,* June 1998, 83(6): 1853–59.

Rosmond, R., G. Holm, and P. Bjorntorp. "Food-Induced Cortisol Secretion in Relation to Anthropometric, Metabolic and Haemodynamic Variables in Men." *International Journal of Obesity and Related Metabolic Disorders,* April 2000, 24(4):416–22.

Sapolsky, R. M., and P. M. Plotsky. "Hypercortisolism and Its Possible Neural Bases." *Biological Psychiatry,* 1 May 1990, 27(9): 937–52.

Sapse, A. T. "Cortisol, High-Cortisol Diseases and Anti-Cortisol Therapy." *Psychoneuroendocrinology,* 1997, 22(suppl. 1): S3–10.

Svec, F., and A. L. Shawar. "The Acute Effect of a Noontime Meal on the Serum Levels of Cortisol and DHEA in Lean and Obese Women." *Psychoneuroendocrinology,* 1997, 22(suppl. 1): S115–19.

Swaab, D. F., F. C. Raadsheer, E. Endert, M. A. Hofman, W. Kamphorst, and R. Ravid. "Increased Cortisol Levels in Aging and Alzheimer's Disease in Postmortem Cerebrospinal Fluid." *Journal of Neuroendocrinology,* December 1994, 6(6): 681–87.

Takahara, J., H. Hosogi, S. Yunoki, K. Hashimoto, and T. Uneki. "Hypothalamic Pituitary Adrenal Function in Patients with Anorexia Nervosa." *Endocrinology-Japan,* December 1976, 23(6): 451–56.

Tsigos, C., R. J. Young, and A. White. "Diabetic Neuropathy Is Associated with Increased Activity of the Hypothalamic-Pituitary-Adrenal Axis." *Journal of Clinical Endocrinology and Metabolism,* March 1993, 76(3): 554–58.

Varma, V. K., J. T. Rushing, and W. H. Ettinger, Jr. "High Density Lipoprotein Cholesterol Is Associated with Serum Cortisol in Older People." *Journal of the American Geriatric Society,* December 1995, 43(12):1345–59.

Vicennati, V., and R. Pasquali. "Abnormalities of the Hypothalamic-Pituitary-Adrenal Axis in Nondepressed Women with Abdominal Obesity and Relations with Insulin Resistance: Evidence for a Central and a

Peripheral Alteration." *Journal of Clinical Endocrinology and Metabolism,* November 2000, 85(11): 4093–98.

Walder, D. J., E. F. Walker, and R. J. Lewine. "Cognitive Functioning, Cortisol Release, and Symptom Severity in Patients with Schizophrenia." *Biological Psychiatry,* 15 December 2000, 48(12): 1121–32.

Walker, B. R., S. Soderberg, B. Lindahl, and T. Olsson. "Independent Effects of Obesity and Cortisol in Predicting Cardiovascular Risk Factors in Men and Women." *Journal of Internal Medicine,* February 2000, 247(2): 198–204.

Weiner, M. F., S. Vobach, D. Svetlik, and R. C. Risser. "Cortisol Secretion and Alzheimer's Disease Progression: A Preliminary Report." *Biological Psychiatry,* 1 August 1993, 34(3): 158–61.

Chapter 4: HSD

Ayachi, S. E., O. Paulmyer-Lacroix, M. Verdier, M. C. Alessi, A. Dutour, and M. Grino. "11 Beta-Hydroxysteroid Dehydrogenase Type 1-Driven Cortisone Reactivation Regulates Plasminogen Activator Inhibitor Type 1 in Adipose Tissue of Obese Women." *Journal of Thrombosis and Haemostasis,* March 2006, 4(3): 621–7.

Basu, R., R. Singh, A. Basu, C. M. Johnson, and R. A. Rizza. "Effect of Nutrient Ingestion on Total-Body and Splanchnic Cortisol Production in Humans." *Diabetes,* March 2006, 55(3): 667–74.

Black, P. H. "The Inflammatory Consequences of Psychologic Stress: Relationship to Insulin Resistance, Obesity, Atherosclerosis and Diabetes Mellitus, Type II." *Medical Hypotheses,* 2006, 67(4): 879–91, E-pub 15 June 2006.

Bobbert, T., L. Brechtel, K. Mai, B. Otto, C. Maser-Gluth, A. F. Pfeiffer, J. Spranger, and S. Diederich. "Adaptation of the Hypothalamic-Pituitary Hormones During Intensive Endurance Training." *Clinical Endocrinology,* November 2005, 63(5): 530–6.

Bujalska, I. J., M. Quinkler, J. W. Tomlinson, C. T. Montague, D. M. Smith, and P. M. Stewart. "Expression Profiling of 11 Beta-Hydroxysteroid Dehydrogenase Type-1 and Glucocorticoid Target Genes in Subcutaneous and Omental Human Preadipocytes." *Journal of Molecular Endocrinology,* October 2006, 37(2): 327–40.

Desbriere, R., V. Vuaroqueaux, V. Achard, S. Boullu-Ciocca, M. Labuhn, A. Dutour, and M. Grino. "11 Beta-Hydroxysteroid Dehydrogenase Type 1 mRNA Is Increased in Both Visceral and Subcutaneous Adipose Tissue of Obese Patients." *Obesity,* May 2006, 14(5): 794–8.

Gambineri, A., V. Vicennati, S. Genghini, F. Tomassoni, U. Pagotto, R. Pasquali, and B. R. Walker. "Genetic Variation in 11 Beta-Hydroxysteroid Dehydrogenase Type 1 Predicts Adrenal Hyperandrogenism among Lean Women with Polycystic Ovary Syndrome." *Journal of Clinical Endocrinology and Metabolism,* June 2006, 91(6): 2295–302, E-pub 21 March 2006.

Koska, J., B. de Courten, D. J. Wake, S. Nair, B. R. Walker, J. C. Bunt, P. A. Permana, R. S. Lindsay, and P. A. Tataranni. "11 Beta-Hydroxysteroid Dehydrogenase Type 1 in Adipose Tissue and Prospective Changes in Body Weight and Insulin Resistance." *Obesity,* September 2006, 14(9): 1515–22.

Mariniello, B., V. Ronconi, S. Rilli, P. Bernante, M. Boscaro, F. Mantero, and G. Giacchetti. "Adipose Tissue 11 Beta-Hydroxysteroid Dehydrogenase Type 1 Expression in Obesity and Cushing's Syndrome." *European Journal of Endocrinology,* September 2006, 155(3): 435–41.

Oppermann, U. "Type 1 11 Beta-Hydroxysteroid Dehydrogenase as Universal Drug Target in Metabolic Diseases?" *Endocrine, Metabolic, and Immune Disorders Drug Targets,* September 2006, 6(3): 259–69.

Paulsen, S. K., S. B. Pedersen, J. O. Jorgensen, S. Fisker, J. S. Christiansen, A. Flyvbjerg, and B. Richelsen. "Growth Hormone (GH) Substitution in GH-Deficient Patients Inhibits 11 Beta-Hydroxysteroid Dehydrogenase Type 1 Messenger Ribonucleic Acid Expression in Adipose Tissue." *Journal of Clinical Endocrinology and Metabolism,* March 2006, 91(3): 1093–8, E-pub 20 December 2005.

Pretorius, E., B. Wallner, and J. Marx. "Cortisol Resistance in Conditions Such as Asthma and the Involvement of 11 Beta-HSD-2: A Hypothesis." *Hormone and Metabolic Research,* June 2006, 38(6): 368–76.

Schuster, D., E. M. Maurer, C. Laggner, L. G. Nashev, T. Wilckens, T. Langer, and A. Odermatt. "The Discovery of New 11 Beta-Hydroxysteroid Dehydrogenase Type 1 Inhibitors by Common Feature Pharmacophore Modeling and Virtual Screening." *Journal of Medicinal Chemistry,* 15 June 2006, 49(12): 3454–66.

Seckl, J. R., and M. J. Meaney. "Glucocorticoid 'Programming' and PTSD Risk." *Annals of the New York Academy of Sciences*, July 2006, 1071: 351–78.

Su, X., N. Vicker, D. Ganeshapillai, A. Smith, A. Purohit, M. J. Reed, and B. V. Potter. "Benzothiazole Derivatives as Novel Inhibitors of Human 11 Beta-Hydroxysteroid Dehydrogenase Type 1." *Molecular and Cellular Endocrinology*, 27 March 2006, 248(1–2): 214–7.

Sukhija, R., P. Kakar, V. Mehta, and J. L. Mehta. "Enhanced 11 Beta-Hydroxysteroid Dehydrogenase Activity, the Metabolic Syndrome, and Systemic Hypertension." *The American Journal of Cardiology*, 15 August 2006, 98(4): 544–8, E-pub 28 June 2006.

Walker, B. R., and R. Andrew. "Tissue Production of Cortisol by 11 Beta-Hydroxysteroid Dehydrogenase Type 1 and Metabolic Disease." *Annals of the New York Academy of Sciences*, November 2006, 1083: 165–84.

Wang, M. "Inhibitors of 11 Beta-Hydroxysteroid Dehydrogenase Type 1 for the Treatment of Metabolic Syndrome." *Current Opinion in Investigational Drugs*, April 2006, 7(4): 319–23.

Chapter 5: Testosterone

Bell, R. J., S. Donath, S. L. Davison, and S. R. Davis. "Endogenous Androgen Levels and Well-Being: Differences Between Premenopausal and Postmenopausal Women." *Menopause*, January–February 2006, 13(1): 65–71.

Chen, R.Y., G. A. Wittert, and G. R. Andrews. "Relative Androgen Deficiency in Relation to Obesity and Metabolic Status in Older Men." *Diabetes, Obesity and Metabolism*, July 2006, 8(4): 429–35.

Cikim, A. S., N. Ozbey, E. Sencer, S. Molvalilar, and Y. Orhan. "Associations among Sex Hormone Binding Globulin Concentrations and Characteristics of the Metabolic Syndrome in Obese Women." *Diabetes, Nutrition and Metabolism*, October 2004, 17(5): 290–5.

Cohen, P. G. "Diabetes Mellitus Is Associated with Subnormal Levels of Free Testosterone in Men." *BJU International*, March 2006, 97(3): 652–3.

Derby, C. A., S. Zilber, D. Brambilla, K. H. Morales, and J. B. McKinlay. "Body Mass Index, Waist Circumference and Waist to Hip Ratio and Change in Sex Steroid Hormones: The Massachusetts Male Aging Study." *Clinical Endocrinology*, July 2006, 65(1): 125–31.

Elin, R. J., and S. J. Winters. "Current Controversies in Testosterone Testing: Aging and Obesity." *Clinical Laboratory Medicine*, March 2004, 24(1): 119–39.

Gapstur, S. M., P. Kopp, P. H. Gann, B. C. Chiu, L. A. Colangelo, and K. Liu. "Changes in BMI Modulate Age-Associated Changes in Sex Hormone Binding Globulin and Total Testosterone, but Not Bioavailable Testosterone in Young Adult Men: The CARDIA Male Hormone Study." *International Journal of Obesity*, Apr. 2007, 31(4): 685–91.

Kaplan, S. A., A. G. Meehan, and A. Shah. "The Age Related Decrease in Testosterone Is Significantly Exacerbated in Obese Men with the Metabolic Syndrome. What Are the Implications for the Relatively High Incidence of Erectile Dysfunction Observed in These Men?" *The Journal of Urology*, October 2006, 176(4 Pt. 1): 1524–7.

Lunenfeld, B. "Endocrinology of the Aging Male." *Minerva Ginecologica*, April. 2006, 58(2): 153–70.

Mayes, J. S., and G. H. Watson. "Direct Effects of Sex Steroid Hormones on Adipose Tissues and Obesity." *Obesity Reviews*, November 2004, 5(4): 197–216.

McTiernan, A., S. S. Tworoger, K. B. Rajan, Y. Yasui, B. Sorenson, C. M. Ulrich, J. Chubak, F. Z. Stanczyk, D. Bowen, M. L. Irwin, R. E. Rudolph, J. D. Potter, and R. S. Schwartz. "Effect of Exercise on Serum Androgens in Postmenopausal Women: A 12-Month Randomized Clinical Trial." *Cancer Epidemiology Biomarkers and Prevention*, July 2004, 13(7): 1099–105.

McTiernan, A., L. Wu, C. Chen, R. Chlebowski, Y. Mossavar-Rahmani, F. Modugno, M. G. Perri, F. Z. Stanczyk, L. Van Horn, C. Y. Wang; Women's Health Initiative Investigators. "Relation of BMI and Physical Activity to Sex Hormones in Postmenopausal Women." *Obesity*, September 2006, 14(9): 1662–77.

Mohr, B. A., S. Bhasin, C. L. Link, A. B. O'Donnell, and J. B. McKinlay. "The Effect of Changes in Adiposity on Testosterone Levels in Older Men: Longitudinal Results from the Massachusetts Male Aging Study." *European Journal of Endocrinology*, September 2006, 155(3): 443–52.

Osuna, J. A., R. Gomez-Perez, G. Arata-Bellabarba, and V. Villaroel. "Relationship Between BMI, Total Testosterone, Sex Hormone-Binding-Globulin, Leptin, Insulin and Insulin Resistance in Obese Men." *Archives of Andrology*, September–October 2006, 52(5): 355–61.

Pasquali, R. "Obesity and Androgens: Facts and Perspectives." *Fertility and Sterility*, May 2006, 85(5): 1319–40.

Travison, T. G., A. B. Araujo, A. B. O'Donnell, V. Kupelian, and J. B. McKinlay. "A Population-Level Decline in Serum Testosterone Levels in American Men." *Journal of Clinical Endocrinology and Metabolism*, January 2007, 92(1): 196–202.

Vicennati, V., L. Ceroni, S. Genghini, L. Patton, U. Pagotto, and R. Pasquali. "Sex Difference in the Relationship Between the Hypothalamic-Pituitary-Adrenal Axis and Sex Hormones in Obesity." *Obesity*, February 2006, 14(2): 235–43.

Chapter 8: Dietary Supplements

Supplements to Avoid

General: Cortisol and Herbal Stimulants

Al'Absi, M., W. R. Lovallo, B. McKey, B. H. Sung, T. L. Whitsett, and M. F. Wilson. "Hypothalamic-Pituitary-Adrenocortical Responses to Psychological Stress and Caffeine in Men at High and Low Risk for Hypertension." *Psychosomatic Medicine*, July–August 1998, 60(4): 521–27.

Charney, D. S., G. R. Heninger, and P. I. Jatlow. "Increased Anxiogenic Effects of Caffeine in Panic Disorders." *Archives of General Psychiatry*, March 1985, 42(3): 233–43.

Gilbert, D. G., W. D. Dibb, L. C. Plath, and S. G. Hiyane. "Effects of Nicotine and Caffeine, Separately and in Combination, on EEG Topography, Mood, Heart Rate, Cortisol, and Vigilance." *Psychophysiology*, September 2000, 37(5): 583–95.

Lovallo, W. R., M. al'Absi, K. Blick, T. L. Whitsett, and M. F. Wilson. "Stress-Like Adrenocorticotropin Responses to Caffeine in Young Healthy Men." *Pharmacology, Biochemistry, and Behavior*, November 1996, 55(3): 365–69.

Lovallo, W. R., G. A. Pincomb, B. H. Sung, R. B. Passey, K. P. Sausen, and M. F. Wilson. "Caffeine May Potentiate Adrenocortical Stress Responses in Hypertension-Prone Men." *Hypertension*, August 1989, 14(2): 170–76.

Mattila, M., T. Seppala, and M. J. Mattila. "Anxiogenic Effect of Yohimbine in Healthy Subjects: Comparison with Caffeine and Antagonism by Clonidine and Diazepam." *International Clinical Psychopharmacology*, July 1988, 3(3): 215–29.

Paquot, N., P. Schneiter, E. Jequier, and L. Tappy. "Effects of Glucocorticoids and Sympathomimetic Agents on Basal and Insulin-Stimulated Glucose Metabolism." *Clinical Physiology*, May 1995, 15(3): 231–40.

Pincomb, G. A., W. R. Lovallo, R. B. Passey, D. J. Brackett, and M. F. Wilson. "Caffeine Enhances the Physiological Response to Occupational Stress in Medical Students." *Health and Psychology*, 1987, 6(2): 101–12.

Shepard, J. D., M. al'Absi, T. L. Whitsett, R. B. Passey, and W. R. Lovallo. "Additive Pressor Effects of Caffeine and Stress in Male Medical Students at Risk for Hypertension." *American Journal of Hypertension*, May 2000, 13 (5, pt. 1): 475–81.

Ephedra/Ma Huang/Sida Cordifolia

Astrup, A., L. Breum, S. Toubro, P. Hein, and F. Quaade. "The Effect and Safety of an Ephedrine/Caffeine Compound Compared to Ephedrine, Caffeine and Placebo in Obese Subjects on an Energy-Restricted Diet: A Double Blind Trial." *International Journal of Obesity and Related Metabolic Disorders*, April 1992, 16(4): 269–77.

Astrup, A., L. Breum, and S. Toubro. "Pharmacological and Clinical Studies of Ephedrine and Other Thermogenic Agonists." *Obesity Research*, November 1995, 3(suppl. 4): S537–40.

Breum. L., J. K. Pedersen, F. Ahlstrom, and J. Frimodt-Moller. "Comparison of an Ephedrine/Caffeine Combination and Dexfenfluramine in the Treatment of Obesity: A Double-Blind Multi-Centre Trial in General Practice." *International Journal of Obesity and Related Metabolic Disorders*, February 1994, 18(2): 99–103.

Daly, P. A., D. R. Krieger, A. G. Dulloo, J. B. Young, and L. Landsberg. "Ephedrine, Caffeine and Aspirin: Safety and Efficacy for Treatment of Human Obesity." *International Journal of Obesity and Related Metabolic Disorders*, February 1993, 17(suppl. 1): S73–78.

Gurley, B. J., S. F. Gardner, and M. A. Hubbard. "Content Versus Label Claims in Ephedra-Containing Dietary Supplements." *American Journal of Health Systems Pharmacology*, 15 May 2000, 57(10): 963–69.

Toubro, S., A. V. Astrup, L. Breum, and F. Quaade. "Safety and Efficacy of Long-Term Treatment with Ephedrine, Caffeine and an Ephedrine/Caffeine Mixture." *International Journal of Obesity and Related Metabolic Disorders*, February 1993, 17(suppl. 1): S69–72.

Toubro. S., A. Astrup, L. Breum, and F. Quaade. "The Acute and Chronic Effects of Ephedrine/Caffeine Mixtures on Energy Expenditure and Glucose Metabolism in Humans." *International Journal of Obesity and Related Metabolic Disorders*, December 1993, 17(suppl. 3): S73–77; discussion S82.

Guarana

Galduroz, J. C., and E. de A. Carlini. "Acute Effects of the Paullinia Cupana 'Guarana' on the Cognition of Normal Volunteers." *Revista Paulista de Medicina*, July–September 1994, 112(3): 607–11.

Galduroz, J. C., and E. de A. Carlini. "The Effects of Long-Term Administration of Guarana on the Cognition of Normal, Elderly Volunteers." *Revista Paulista de Medicina*, January–February 1996, 114(1): 1073–78.

Katzung, W. "Guarana: A Natural Product with High Caffeine Content." *Medizinische Monatsschrift Pharmazeuten*, November 1993, 16(11): 330–33.

Synephrine/Zhi Shi/Citrus Aurantium

Chen, X., L. Y. Liu, H. W. Deng, Y. X. Fang, and Y. W. Ye. "The Effects of Citrus Aurantium and Its Active Ingredient N-Methyltyramine on the Cardiovascular Receptors." *Yao Hsueh Hsueh Pao*, April 1981, 16(4): 253–59.

Fontana, E., N. Morin, D. Prevot, and C. Carpene. "Effects of Octopamine on Lipolysis, Glucose Transport and Amine Oxidation in Mammalian Fat Cells." *Comparative Biochemistry and Physiology. Toxicology and Pharmacology*, January 2000, 125(1): 33–44.

Galitzky, J., C. Carpene, M. Lafontan, and M. Berlan. "Specific Stimulation of Adipose Tissue Adrenergic Beta 3 Receptors by Octopamine." *Comptes Rendus de l'Academie des Sciences. Serie III, Sciences de la Vie*, 1993, 316(5): 519–23.

Yohimbe/Quebracho

Adimoelja, A. "Phytochemicals and the Breakthrough of Traditional Herbs in the Management of Sexual Dysfunctions." *International Journal of Andrology*, 2000, 23(suppl. 2): 82–84.

De Smet, P. A., and O. S. Smeets. "Potential Risks of Health-Food Products Containing Yohimbe Extracts." *British Medical Journal*, 8 October 1994, 309(6959): 958.

Coleus

Greenway, F. L., and G. A. Bray. "Regional Fat Loss from the Thigh in Obese Women after Adrenergic Modulation." *Clinical Therapy*, 1987, 9(6): 663–69.

Martin, L. F., C. M. Klim, S. J. Vannucci, L. B. Dixon, J. R. Landis, and K. F. LaNoue. "Alterations in Adipocyte Adenylate Cyclase Activity in Morbidly Obese and Formerly Morbidly Obese Humans." *Surgery*, August 1990, 108(2): 228–34; discussion 234–35.

Mauriege, P., D. Prud'homme, S. Lemieux, A. Tremblay, and J. P. Despres. "Regional Differences in Adipose Tissue Lipolysis from Lean and Obese Women: Existence of Postreceptor Alterations." *American Journal of Physiology*, August 1995, 269(2, pt. 1): E341–50.

Mauriege, P., D. Prud'homme, M. Marcotte, M. Yoshioka, A. Tremblay, and J. P. Despres. "Regional Differences in Adipose Tissue Metabolism Between Sedentary and Endurance-Trained Women." *American Journal of Physiology*, September 1997, 273(3, pt. 1): E497–506.

Van Belle, H. "Is There a Role for cAMP and Adenyl Cyclase?" *Journal of Cardiovascular Pharmacology*, 1985, 7(suppl. 5): S28–32.

Vitamins and Minerals for Stress Adaptation

Vitamin C

Halliwell, B. "Antioxidant Defense Mechanisms: From the Beginning to the End (of the Beginning)." *Free-Radical Research*, October 1999, 31(4): 261–72.

Jacob, R. A., F. S. Pianalto, and R. E. Agee. "Cellular Ascorbate Depletion in Healthy Men." *Journal of Nutrition*, May 1992, 122(5): 1111–18.

Johnston, C. S., C. G. Meyer, and J. C. Srilakshmi. "Vitamin C Elevates Red Blood Cell Glutathione in Healthy Adults." *American Journal of Clinical Nutrition*, July 1993, 58(1): 103–5.

Rokitzki, L., S. Hinkel, C. Klemp, D. Cufi, and J. Keul. "Dietary, Serum and Urine Ascorbic Acid Status in Male Athletes." *International Journal of Sports Medicine*, October 1994, 15(7): 435–40.

Sinclair, A. J., P. B. Taylor, J. Lunec, A. J. Girling, and A. H. Barnett. "Low Plasma Ascorbate Levels in Patients with Type-2 Diabetes Mellitus Consuming Adequate Dietary Vitamin C." *Diabetes Medicine*, November 1994, 11(9): 893–98.

VanderJagt, D. J., P. J. Garry, and H. N. Bhagavan. "Ascorbic Acid Intake and Plasma Levels in Healthy Elderly People." *American Journal of Clinical Nutrition*, August 1987, 46(2): 290–94.

Calcium

Heaney, R. P. "Low Calcium Intake among African Americans: Effects on Bones and Body Weight." *Journal of Nutrition*, April 2006, 136(4): 1095–8.

Major, G. C., F. Alarie, J. Dore, S. Phouttama, and A. Tremblay. "Supplementation with Calcium + Vitamin D Enhances the Beneficial Effect of Weight Loss on Plasma Lipid and Lipoprotein Concentrations." *American Journal of Clinical Nutrition*, January 2007, 85(1): 54–9.

Zemel, M. B. "The Role of Dairy Foods in Weight Management." *Journal of the American College of Nutrition*, December 2005, 24(6 Suppl): 537S–46S.

Zemel, M. B., J. Richards, A. Milstead, and P. Campbell. "Effects of Calcium and Dairy on Body Composition and Weight Loss in African-American Adults." *Obesity Research*, Jul. 2005, 13(7): 1218–25.

Magnesium

Altura, B. M., and B. T. Altura. "New Perspectives on the Role of Magnesium in the Pathophysiology of the Cardiovascular System: Clinical Aspects." *Magnesium*, 1985, 4(5-6): 226–44.

Paddle, B. M., and N. Haugaard. "Role of Magnesium in Effects of Epinephrine on Heart Contraction and Metabolism." *American Journal of Physiology*, October 1971, 221(4): 1178–84.

Savabi, F., V. Gura, S. Bessman, and N. Brautbar. "Effects of Magnesium Depletion on Myocardial High-Energy Phosphates and Contractility." *Biochemical Medicine and Metabolic Biology*, April 1988, 39(2): 131–39.

Zimmermann, P., U. Weiss, H. G. Classen, B. Wendt, A. Epple, H. Zollner, W. Temmel, M. Weger, and S. Porta. "The Impact of Diets with Different Magnesium Contents on Magnesium and Calcium in Serum and Tissues of the Rat." *Life Sciences*, 14 July 2000, 67(8): 949–58.

B-Complex Vitamins (Thiamin, Riboflavin, Pantothenic Acid, Pyridoxine)

Baldewicz, T., K. Goodkin, D. J. Feaster, N. T. Blaney, M. Kumar, A. Kumar, G. Shor-Posner, and M. Baum. "Plasma Pyridoxine Deficiency Is Related to Increased Psychological Distress in Recently Bereaved Homosexual Men." *Psychosomatic Medicine,* May–June 1998, 60(3): 297–308.

Bendich, A. "The Potential for Dietary Supplements to Reduce Premenstrual Syndrome (PMS) Symptoms." *Journal of the American College of Nutrition,* February 2000, 19(1): 3–12.

Bigazzi, M., S. Ferraro, R. Ronga, G. Scarselli, V. Bruni, and A. L. Olivotti. "Effect of Vitamin B-6 on the Serum Concentration of Pituitary Hormones in Normal Humans and under Pathologic Conditions." *Journal of Endocrinological Investigation,* April–June 1979, 2(2): 117–24.

Heap, L. C., T. J. Peters, and S. Wessely. "Vitamin B Status in Patients with Chronic Fatigue Syndrome." *Journal of the Royal Society of Medicine,* April 1999, 92(4): 183–85.

Kopp-Woodroffe, S. A., M. M. Manore, C. A. Dueck, J. S. Skinner, and K. S. Matt. "Energy and Nutrient Status of Amenorrheic Athletes Participating in a Diet and Exercise Training Intervention Program." *International Journal of Sport Nutrition,* March 1999, 9(1): 70–88.

Leung, L. H. "Pantothenic Acid as a Weight-Reducing Agent: Fasting Without Hunger, Weakness and Ketosis." *Medical Hypotheses,* May 1995, 44(5): 403–5.

Manore, M. M. "Effect of Physical Activity on Thiamine, Riboflavin, and Vitamin B-6 Requirements." *American Journal of Clinical Nutrition,* August 2000, 72(2, suppl.): S598–606.

Cortisol-Control Supplements

Magnolia Bark

Kuribara, H., E. Kishi, N. Hattori, M. Okada, and Y. Maruyama. "The Anxiolytic Effect of Two Oriental Herbal Drugs in Japan Attributed to Honokiol from Magnolia Bark." *Journal of Pharmacy and Pharmacology,* November 2000, 52(11): 1425–29.

Wang, S. M., L. J. Lee, Y. T. Huang, J. J. Chen, and Y. L. Chen. "Magnolol Stimulates Steroidogenesis in Rat Adrenal Cells." *British Journal of Pharmacology,* November 2000, 131(6): 1172–78.

Watanabe, K., Y. Goto, and K. Yoshitomi. "Central Depressant Effects of the Extracts of Magnolia Cortex." *Chemical and Pharmacological Bulletin.* Tokyo, August 1973, 21(8): 1700–8.

Watanabe, K., H. Watanabe, Y. Goto, M. Yamaguchi, N. Yamamoto, and K. Hagino. "Pharmacological Properties of Magnolol and Honokiol Extracted from Magnolia Officinalis: Central Depressant Effects." *Planta Medica*, October 1983, 49: 103–8.

Watanabe, K., H. Y. Watanabe, Y. Goto, N. Yamamoto, and M. Yoshizaki. "Studies on the Active Principles of Magnolia Bark: Centrally Acting Muscle Relaxant Activity of Magnolol and Honokiol." *Japanese Journal of Pharmacology*, October 1975, 25(5): 605–7.

Theanine

Kakuda, T., A. Nozawa, T. Unno, N. Okamura, and O. Okai. "Inhibiting Effects of Theanine on Caffeine Stimulation Evaluated by EEG in the Rat." *Biosciences, Biotechnology, and Biochemistry*, February 2000, 64(2): 287–93.

Yokogoshi, H., Y. Kato, Y. M. Sagesaka, T. Takihara-Matsuura, T. Kakuda, and N. Takeuchi. "Reduction Effect of Theanine on Blood Pressure and Brain 5-Hydroxyindoles in Spontaneously Hypertensive Rats." *Biosciences, Biotechnology, and Biochemistry*, April 1995, 59(4): 615–18.

Yokogoshi, H., and T. Terashima. "Effect of Theanine, R-Glutamylethylamide, on Brain Monoamines, Striatal Dopamine Release and Some Kinds of Behavior in Rats." *Nutrition*, September 2000, 16(9): 776–77.

Epimedium

Cai, D., S. Shen, and X. Chen. "Clinical and Experimental Research of Epimedium Brevicornum in Relieving Neuroendocrino-Immunological Effect Inhibited by Exogenous Glucocorticoid." *Zhongguo Zhong Xi Yi Jie He Za Zhi*, January 1998, 18(1): 4–7.

Kuang, A. K., J. L. Chen, and M. D. Chen. "Effects of Yang-Restoring Herb Medicines on the Levels of Plasma Corticosterone, Testosterone and Triiodothyronine." *Zhong Xi Yi Jie He Za Zhi*, December 1989, 9(12): 737–38, 710.

Zhang, J. Q. "Clinical and Experimental Studies on Yang Deficiency." *Journal of Traditional Chinese Medicine*, September 1982, 2(3): 237–42.

Zhong, L. Y., Z. Y. Shen, and D. F. Cai. "Effect of Three Kinds (Tonifying Kidney, Invigorating Spleen, Promoting Blood Circulation) Recipes on the Hypothalamus-Pituitary-Adrenal-Thymus (HPAT) Axis and CRF Gene Expression." *Zhongguo Zhong Xi Yi Jie He Za Zhi*, January 1997, 17(1): 39–41.

Phytosterols

Agren, J. J., E. Tvrzicka, M. T. Nenonen, T. Helve, and O. Hanninen. "Divergent Changes in Serum Sterols During a Strict Uncooked Vegan Diet in Patients with Rheumatoid Arthritis." *British Journal of Nutrition,* February 2001, 85(2): 137–39.

Bouic, P. J., and J. H. Lamprecht. "Plant Sterols and Sterolins: A Review of Their Immune-Modulating Properties." *Alternative Medicine Review,* June 1999, 4(3): 170–77.

"Plant Sterols and Sterolins." *Alternative Medicine Review,* April 2001, 6(2): 203–6.

Phosphatidylserine

Diboune, M., G. Ferard, Y. Ingenbleek, A. Bourguignat, D. Spielmann, C. Scheppler-Roupert, P. A. Tulasne, B. Calon, M. Hasselmann, P. Sauder, et al. "Soybean Oil, Blackcurrant Seed Oil, Medium-Chain Triglycerides, and Plasma Phospholipid Fatty Acids of Stressed Patients." *Nutrition,* July–August 1993, 9(4): 344–49.

Leathwood, P. D. "Neurotransmitter Precursors and Brain Function." *Bibliotheca Nutritio et Dieta,* 1986, (38): 54–71.

Monteleone, P., L. Beinat, C. Tanzillo, M. Maj, and D. Kemali. "Effects of Phosphatidylserine on the Neuroendocrine Response to Physical Stress in Humans." *Neuroendocrinology,* September 1990, 52(3): 243–58.

Monteleone, P., M. Maj, L. Beinat, M. Natale, and D. Kemali. "Blunting by Chronic Phosphatidylserine Administration of the Stress-Induced Activation of the Hypothalamo-Pituitary-Adrenal Axis in Healthy Men." *European Journal of Clinical Pharmacology,* 1992, 42(4): 385–88.

Wurtman, R. J. "Nutrients that Modify Brain Function." *Scientific American,* April 1982, 246(4): 50–9.

Tyrosine

Acworth, I. N., M. J. During, and R. J. Wurtman. "Tyrosine: Effects on Catecholamine Release." *Brain Research Bulletin,* September 1988, 21(3): 473–77.

Caballero, B., R. E. Gleason, and R. J. Wurtman. "Plasma Amino Acid Concentrations in Healthy Elderly Men and Women." *American Journal of Clinical Nutrition,* May 1991, 53(5): 1249–52.

Conlay, L. A., R. J. Wurtman, G. Lopez, I. Coviella, J. K. Blusztajn, C. A. Vacanti, M. Logue, M. During, B. Caballero, T. J. Maher, and G. Evoniuk. "Effects of Running the Boston Marathon on Plasma Concentrations of Large Neutral Amino Acids." *Journal of Neural Transmission*, 1989, 76(1): 65–71.

Dollins, A. B., L. P. Krock, W. F. Storm, R. J. Wurtman, and H. R. Lieberman. "L-Tyrosine Ameliorates Some Effects of Lower Body Negative Pressure Stress." *Physiology and Behavior*, February 1995, 57(2): 223–30.

Lieberman, H. R., S. Corkin, B. J. Spring, R. J. Wurtman, and J. H. Growdon. "The Effects of Dietary Neurotransmitter Precursors on Human Behavior." *American Journal of Clinical Nutrition*, August 1985, 42(2): 366–70.

Milner, J. D., and R. J. Wurtman. "Tyrosine Availability: A Presynaptic Factor Controlling Catecholamine Release." *Advances in Experimental Medicine and Biology*, 1987, 221: 211–21.

Reinstein, D. K., H. Lehnert, and R. J. Wurtman. "Dietary Tyrosine Suppresses the Rise in Plasma Corticosterone Following Acute Stress in Rats." *Life Sciences*, 9 December 1985, 37(23): 2157–63.

Wurtman, R. J. "Effects of Their Nutrient Precursors on the Synthesis and Release of Serotonin, the Catecholamines, and Acetylcholine: Implications for Behavioral Disorders." *Clinical Neuropharmacology*, 1988, 11(suppl. 1): S187–93.

Branched-Chain Amino Acids (BCAAs: Valine, Leucine, and Isoleucine)

Blomstrand, E., F. Celsing, and E. A. Newsholme. "Changes in Plasma Concentrations of Aromatic and Branched-Chain Amino Acids During Sustained Exercise in Man and Their Possible Role in Fatigue." *Acta Physiologica Scandinavia*, May 1988, 133(1): 115–21.

Blomstrand, E., P. Hassmen, S. Ek, B. Ekblom, and E. A. Newsholme. "Influence of Ingesting a Solution of Branched-Chain Amino Acids on Perceived Exertion During Exercise." *Acta Physiologica Scandinavia*, January 1997, 159(1): 41–49.

Castell, L. M., T. Yamamoto, J. Phoenix, and E. A. Newsholme. "The Role of Tryptophan in Fatigue in Different Conditions of Stress." *Advances in Experimental Medicine and Biology*, 1999, 467: 697–704.

Davis, J. M., R. S. Welsh, K. L. De Volve, and N. A. Alderson. "Effects of Branched-Chain Amino Acids and Carbohydrate on Fatigue During Intermittent, High-Intensity Running." *International Journal of Sports Medicine,* July 1999, 20(5): 309–14.

Gastmann, U. A., and M. J. Lehmann. "Overtraining and the BCAA Hypothesis." *Medicine and Science in Sports and Exercise,* July 1998, 30(7): 1173–78.

Hassmen, P., E. Blomstrand, B. Ekblom, and E. A. Newsholme. "Branched-Chain Amino Acid Supplementation During 30-Km Competitive Run: Mood and Cognitive Performance." *Nutrition,* September–October 1994, 10(5): 405–10.

Lehmann, M., M. Huonker, F. Dimeo, N. Heinz, U. Gastmann, N. Treis, J. M. Steinacker, J. Keul, R. Kajewski, and D. Haussinger. "Serum Amino Acid Concentrations in Nine Athletes Before and After the 1993 Colmar Ultra Triathlon." *International Journal of Sports Medicine,* April 1995, 16(3): 155–69.

Mittleman, K. D., M. R. Ricci, and S. P. Bailey. "Branched-Chain Amino Acids Prolong Exercise During Heat Stress in Men and Women." *Medicine and Science in Sports and Exercise,* January 1998, 30(1): 83–91.

Testosterone-Control Supplements

DHEA (Dehydroepiandrosterone)

Brown, G. A., M. D. Vukovich, R. L. Sharp, T. A. Reifenrath, K. A. Parsons, and D. S. King. "Effect of Oral DHEA on Serum Testosterone and Adaptations to Resistance Training in Young Men." *Journal of Applied Physiology,* December 1999, 87(6): 2274–83.

Filaire, E., P. Duche, and G. Lac. "Effects of Amount of Training on the Saliva Concentrations of Cortisol, Dehydroepiandrosterone and on the Dehydroepiandrosterone: Cortisol Concentration Ratio in Women over 16 Weeks of Training." *European Journal of Applied Physiology and Occupational Physiology,* October 1998, 78(5): 466–71.

Filaire, E., P. Duche, and G. Lac. "Effects of Training for Two Ball Games on the Saliva Response of Adrenocortical Hormones to Exercise in Elite Sportswomen." *European Journal of Applied Physiology and Occupational Physiology,* April 1998, 77(5): 452–56.

Keizer, H., G. M. Janssen, P. Menheere, and G. Kranenburg. "Changes in Basal Plasma Testosterone, Cortisol, and Dehydroepiandrosterone Sulfate in Previously Untrained Males and Females Preparing for a Marathon." *International Journal of Sports Medicine*, October 1989, 10(suppl. 3): S139–45.

Zinc

Abbasi, A. A., A. S. Prasad, P. Rabbani, and E. DuMouchelle. "Experimental Zinc Deficiency in Man: Effect on Testicular Function." *Journal of Laboratory and Clinical Medicine*, September 1980, 96(3): 544–50.

Lukaski, H. C. "Magnesium, Zinc, and Chromium Nutriture and Physical Activity." *American Journal of Clinical Nutrition*, August 2000, 72(2, suppl.): S585–93.

McDonald, R., and C. L. Keen. "Iron, Zinc, and Magnesium Nutrition and Athletic Performance." *Sports Medicine*, March 1988, 5(3): 171–84.

Nishi Y. "Anemia and Zinc Deficiency in the Athlete." *Journal of the American College of Nutrition*, August 1996, 15(4): 323–24.

Prasad, A. S. "Zinc Deficiency in Human Subjects." *Progress in Clinical and Biological Research*, 1983, 129: 1–33.

Cordyceps

Bao, T. T., G. F. Wang, and Y. L. Yang. "Pharmacological Actions of Cordyceps Sinensis." *Chung Hsi I Chieh Ho Tsa Chih*, June 1988, 8(6): 352–54, 325–26.

Kuo, Y. C., W. J. Tsai, M. S. Shiao, C. F. Chen, and C. Y. Lin. "Cordyceps Sinensis as an Immunomodulatory Agent." *American Journal of Chinese Medicine*, 1996, 24(2): 111–25.

Zhu, J. S., G. M. Halpern, and K. Jones. "The Scientific Rediscovery of an Ancient Chinese Herbal Medicine: Cordyceps Sinensis: Part I." *Journal of Alternative and Complementary Medicine*, Fall 1998, 4(3): 289–303.

Zhu, J. S., G. M. Halpern, and K. Jones. "The Scientific Rediscovery of a Precious Ancient Chinese Herbal Regimen: Cordyceps Sinensis: Part II." *Journal of Alternative and Complementary Medicine*, Winter 1998, 4(4): 429–57.

Conjugated Linoleic Acid (CLA)

Stangl, G. I. "Conjugated Linoleic Acids Exhibit a Strong Fat-to-Lean Partitioning Effect, Reduce Serum VLDL Lipids and Redistribute Tissue Lipids in Food-Restricted Rats." *Journal of Nutrition*, May 2000, 130(5): 1140–46.

Zambell, K. L., N. L. Keim, M. D. Van Loan, B. Gale, P. Benito, D. S. Kelley, and G. J. Nelson. "Conjugated Linoleic Acid Supplementation in Humans: Effects on Body Composition and Energy Expenditure." *Lipids,* July 2000, 35(7): 777–82.

HMB (Hydroxymethylbutyrate)

Kreider, R. B., M. Ferreira, M. Wilson, and A. L. Almada. "Effects of Calcium Beta-Hydroxy-Beta-Methylbutyrate (HMB) Supplementation During Resistance-Training on Markers of Catabolism, Body Composition and Strength." *International Journal of Sports Medicine,* November 1999, 20(8): 503–9.

Nissen, S., R. Sharp, M. Ray, J. A. Rathmacher, D. Rice, J. C. Fuller, Jr., A. S. Connelly, and N. Abumrad. "Effect of Leucine Metabolite Beta-Hydroxy-Beta-Methylbutyrate on Muscle Metabolism During Resistance-Exercise Training." *Journal of Applied Physiology,* November 1996, 81(5): 2095–104.

Panton, L. B., J. A. Rathmacher, S. Baier, and S. Nissen. "Nutritional Supplementation of the Leucine Metabolite Beta-Hydroxy-Beta-Methylbutyrate (HMB) During Resistance Training." *Nutrition,* Sept. 2000, 16(9): 734–39.

Slater, G. J., and D. Jenkins. "Beta-Hydroxy-Beta-Methylbutyrate (HMB) Supplementation and the Promotion of Muscle Growth and Strength." *Sports Medicine,* August 2000, 30(2): 105–16.

Adaptogens (General Antistress Supplements)

Ginseng

Avakian, E. V., R. B. Sugimoto, S. Taguchi, and S. M. Horvath. "Effect of Panax Ginseng Extract on Energy Metabolism During Exercise in Rats." *Planta Medica,* April 1984, 50(2): 151–54.

Dowling, E. A., D. R. Redondo, J. D. Branch, S. Jones, G. McNabb, and M. H. Williams. "Effect of Eleutherococcus Senticosus on Submaximal and Maximal Exercise Performance." *Medical Science, Sports, and Exercise,* April 1996, 28(4): 482–89.

Wang, B. X., J. C. Cui, A. J. Liu, and S. K. Wu. "Studies on the Anti-Fatigue Effect of the Saponins of Stems and Leaves of Panax Ginseng (SSLG)." *Journal of Traditional Chinese Medicine,* June 1983, 3(2): 89–94.

Wang, L. C., and T. F. Lee. "Effect of Ginseng Saponins on Exercise Performance in Non-Trained Rats." *Planta Medica,* March 1998, 64(2): 130–33.

Ziemba, A. W., J. Chmura, H. Kaciuba-Uscilko, K. Nazar, P. Wisnik, and W. Gawronski. "Ginseng Treatment Improves Psychomotor Performance at Rest and During Graded Exercise in Young Athletes." *International Journal of Sport Nutrition*, December 1999, 9(4): 371–77.

Ashwagandha

Bhattacharya, S. K., A. Bhattacharya, K. Sairam, and S. Ghosal. "Anxiolytic-Antidepressant Activity of Withania Somnifera Glycowith-anolides: An Experimental Study." *Phytomedicine*, December 2000, 7(6): 463–69.

Dhuley, J. N. "Adaptogenic and Cardioprotective Action of Ashwagandha in Rats and Frogs." *Journal of Ethnopharmacology*, April 2000, 70(1): 57–63.

Dhuley, J. N. "Effect of Ashwagandha on Lipid Peroxidation in Stress-Induced Animals." *Journal of Ethnopharmacology*, March 1998, 60(2): 173–78.

Mishra, L. C., B. B. Singh, and S. Dagenais. "Scientific Basis for the Therapeutic Use of Withania Somnifera (Ashwagandha): A Review." *Alternative Medicine Review*, August 2000, 5(4): 334–46.

Ziauddin, M., N. Phansalkar, P. Patki, S. Diwanay, and B. Patwardhan. "Studies on the Immunomodulatory Effects of Ashwagandha." *Journal of Ethnopharmacology*, February 1996, 50(2): 69–76.

Suma

Arletti, R., A. Benelli, E. Cavazzuti, G. Scarpetta, and A. Bertolini. "Stimulating Property of Turnera Diffusa and Pfaffia Paniculata Extracts on the Sexual Behavior of Male Rats." *Psychopharmacology*. Berlin, March 1999, 143(1): 15–19.

Watanabe, T., M. Watanabe, Y. Watanabe, and C. Hotta. "Effects of Oral Administration of Pfaffia Paniculata (Brazilian Ginseng) on Incidence of Spontaneous Leukemia in AKR/J Mice." *Cancer Detection and Prevention*, 2000, 24(2): 173–78.

Schisandra

Li, P. C., K. T. Poon, and K. M. Ko. "Schisandra Chinensis-Dependent Myocardial Protective Action of Sheng-Mai-San in Rats." *American Journal of Chinese Medicine*, 1996, 24(3-4): 255–62.

Liu, G. T. "Advances in Research of the Action of Components Isolated from Fructus Schizandrae Chinensis on Animal Livers." *Chung Hsi I Chieh Ho Tsa Chih*, May 1983, 3(3): 182–85.

Yan-yong, C., S. Zeng-bao, and L. Lian-niang. "Studies of Fructus Schizandrae IV: Isolation and Determination of the Active Compounds (in Lowering High SGPT Levels) of Schizandra Chinensis." *Baillieres Scientifica Sinica.* March–April 1976, 19(2): 276–90.

Rhodiola

Maslova, L. V., B. Iu. Kondrat'ev, L. N. Maslov, and Iu. B. Lishmanov. "The Cardioprotective and Antiadrenergic Activity of an Extract of Rhodiola Rosea in Stress." *Eksperimental Klinicheskaia Farmakologiia,* November–December 1994, 57(6): 61–63.

Rege, N. N., U. M. Thatte, and S. A. Dahanukar. "Adaptogenic Properties of Six Rasayana Herbs Used in Ayurvedic Medicine." *Phytotherapy Research,* June 1999, 13(4): 275–91.

Spasov, A. A., G. K. Wikman, V. B. Mandrikov, I. A. Mironova, and V. V. Neumoin. "A Double-Blind, Placebo-Controlled Pilot Study of the Stimulating and Adaptogenic Effect of Rhodiola Rosea SHR-5 Extract on the Fatigue of Students Caused by Stress During an Examination Period with a Repeated Low-Dose Regimen." *Phytomedicine,* April 2000, 7(2): 85–89.

Astragalus

Sinclair, S. "Chinese Herbs: A Clinical Review of Astragalus, Ligusticum, and Schizandrae." *Alternative Medicine Review,* October 1998, 3(5): 338–44.

Sugiura, H., H. Nishida, R. Inaba, and H. Iwata. "Effects of Exercise in the Growing Stage in Mice and of Astragalus Membranaceus on Immune Functions." *Nippon Eiseigaku Zasshi,* February 1993, 47(6): 1021–31.

Sun, Y., E. M. Hersh, M. Talpaz, S. L. Lee, W. Wong, T. L. Loo, and G. M. Mavligit. "Immune Restoration and/or Augmentation of Local Graft Versus Host Reaction by Traditional Chinese Medicinal Herbs." *Cancer,* 1 July 1983, 52(1): 70–73.

Zhao, K. S., C. Mancini, and G. Doria. "Enhancement of the Immune Response in Mice by Astragalus Membranaceus Extracts." *Immunopharmacology,* November–December 1990, 20(3): 225–33.

Relaxation and Calming Supplements

Kava Kava

Heiligenstein, E., and G. Guenther. "Over-the-Counter Psychotropics: A Review of Melatonin, St. John's Wort, Valerian, and Kava-Kava." *Journal of the American College of Health,* May 1998, 46(6): 271–76.

Herberg, K. W. "Effect of Kava-Special Extract WS 1490 Combined with Ethyl Alcohol on Safety-Relevant Performance Parameters." *Blutalkohol,* March 1993, 30(2): 96–105.

Muller, B., and R. Komorek. "Treatment with Kava: The Root to Combat Stress." *Wiener Medzinische Wochenschrift,* 1999, 149(8–10): 197–201.

Pittler, M. H., and E. Ernst. "Efficacy of Kava Extract for Treating Anxiety: Systematic Review and Meta-Analysis." *Journal of Clinical Psychopharmacology,* February 2000, 20(1): 84–89.

Scherer, J. "Kava-Kava Extract in Anxiety Disorders: An Outpatient Observational Study." *Advances in Therapy.* July–August 1998, 15(4): 261–69.

Volz, H. P., and M. Kieser. "Kava-Kava Extract WS 1490 Versus Placebo in Anxiety Disorders: A Randomized Placebo-Controlled 25-Week Outpatient Trial." *Pharmacopsychiatry,* January 1997, 30(1): 1–5.

Melatonin

Arendt, J., and S. Deacon. "Treatment of Circadian Rhythm Disorders: Melatonin." *Chronobiology International,* March 1997, 14(2): 185–204.

Chase, J. E., and B. E. Gidal. "Melatonin: Therapeutic Use in Sleep Disorders." *Annals of Pharmacotherapy,* October 1997, 31(10): 1218–26.

Defrance, R., and M. A. Quera-Salva. "Therapeutic Applications of Melatonin and Related Compounds." *Hormone Research,* 1998, 49(3–4): 142–46.

Jan, J. E., H. Espezel, R. D. Freeman, and D. K. Fast. "Melatonin Treatment of Chronic Sleep Disorders." *Journal of Childhood Neurology,* February 1998, 13(2): 98.

Okawa, M., M. Uchiyama, S. Ozaki, K. Shibui, Y. Kamei, T. Hayakawa, and J. Urata. "Melatonin Treatment for Circadian Rhythm Sleep Disorders." *Psychiatry and Clinical Neuroscience,* April 1998, 52(2): 259–60.

Sack, R. L., R. J. Hughes, D. M. Edgar, and A. J. Lewy. "Sleep-Promoting Effects of Melatonin: At What Dose, in Whom, under What Conditions, and by What Mechanisms?" *Sleep,* October 1997, 20(10): 908–15.

Sack, R. L., A. J. Lewy, and R. J. Hughes. "Use of Melatonin for Sleep and Circadian Rhythm Disorders." *Annals of Medicine,* February 1998, 30(1): 115–21.

Valerian

Balderer, G., and A. A. Borbely. "Effect of Valerian on Human Sleep." *Psychopharmacology*, Berlin, 1985, 87(4): 406–9.

Donath, F., S. Quispe, K. Diefenbach, A. Maurer, I. Fietze, and I. Roots. "Critical Evaluation of the Effect of Valerian Extract on Sleep Structure and Sleep Quality." *Pharmacopsychiatry*, March 2000, 33(2): 47–53.

Houghton, P. J. "The Biological Activity of Valerian and Related Plants." *Journal of Ethnopharmacology*, February–March, 1988, 22(2): 121–42.

Schmitz, M., and M. Jackel. "Comparative Study for Assessing Quality of Life of Patients with Exogenous Sleep Disorders (Temporary Sleep Onset and Sleep Interruption Disorders) Treated with a Hops-Valerian Preparation and a Benzodiazepine Drug." *Wiener Medizinische Wochen-schrift*, 1998, 148(13): 291–98.

Gotu Kola

Bradwejn, J., Y. Zhou, D. Koszycki, and J. Shlik. "A Double-Blind, Placebo-Controlled Study on the Effects of Gotu Kola (Centella Asiatica) on Acoustic Startle Response in Healthy Subjects." *Journal of Clinical Psychopharmacology*, December 2000, 20(6): 680–84.

Shukla, A., A. M. Rasik, and B. N. Dhawan. "Asiaticoside-Induced Elevation of Antioxidant Levels in Healing Wounds." *Phytotherapy Research*, February 1999, 13(1): 50–54.

St. John's Wort

De Vry, J., S. Maurel, R. Schreiber, R. de Beun, and K. R. Jentzsch. "Comparison of Hypericum Extracts with Imipramine and Fluoxetine in Animal Models of Depression and Alcoholism." *European Neuropsychopharmacology*, December 1999, 9(6): 461–68.

Gaster, B., and J. Holroyd. "St John's Wort for Depression: A Systematic Review." *Archives of Internal Medicine*, 24 January 2000, 160(2): 152–56.

Hansgen, K. D., J. Vesper, and M. Ploch. "Multicenter Double-Blind Study Examining the Antidepressant Effectiveness of the Hypericum Extract LI 160." *Journal of Geriatric Psychiatry and Neurology*, October 1994, 7(suppl. 1): S15–18.

Hubner, W. D., S. Lande, and H. Podzuweit. "Hypericum Treatment of Mild Depressions with Somatic Symptoms." *Journal of Geriatric Psychiatry and Neurology*, October 1994, 7(suppl. 1): S12–14.

Kasper S. "Treatment of Seasonal Affective Disorder (SAD) with Hypericum Extract." *Pharmacopsychiatry*, September 1997, 30(suppl. 2): 89–93.

Laakmann, G., C. Schule, T. Baghai, and M. Kieser. "St. John's Wort in Mild to Moderate Depression: The Relevance of Hyperforin for the Clinical Efficacy." *Pharmacopsychiatry*, June 1998, 31(suppl. 1): 54–59.

Linde, K., G. Ramirez, C. D. Mulrow, A. Pauls, W. Weidenhammer, and D. Melchart. "St. John's Wort for Depression: An Overview and Meta-Analysis of Randomised Clinical Trials." *British Medical Journal*, 3 August 1996, 313(7052): 253–58.

Miller, A. L. "St. John's Wort (Hypericum Perforatum): Clinical Effects on Depression and Other Conditions." *Alternative Medicine Review*, February 1998, 3(1): 18–26.

Stevinson, C., and E. Ernst. "Hypericum for Depression: An Update of the Clinical Evidence." *European Neuropsychopharmacology*, December 1999, 9(6): 501–5.

Volz, H. P., and P. Laux. "Potential Treatment for Subthreshold and Mild Depression: A Comparison of St. John's Wort Extracts and Fluoxetine." *Comprehensive Psychiatry*, March–April 2000, 41(2, suppl. 1): 133–37.

5-Hydroxytryptophan (5-HTP)

Birdsall, T. C. "5-Hydroxytryptophan: A Clinically-Effective Serotonin Precursor." *Alternative Medicine Review*, August 1998, 3(4): 271–80.

Byerley, W. F., L. L. Judd, F. W. Reimherr, and B. I. Grosser. "5-Hydroxytryptophan: A Review of Its Antidepressant Efficacy and Adverse Effects." *Journal of Clinical Psychopharmacology*, June 1987, 7(3): 127–37.

Cangiano, C., A. Laviano, M. Del Ben, I. Preziosa, F. Angelico, A. Cascino, and F. Rossi-Fanelli. "Effects of Oral 5-Hydroxy-Tryptophan on Energy Intake and Macronutrient Selection in Non-Insulin-Dependent Diabetic Patients." *International Journal of Obesity and Related Metabolic Disorders*, July 1998, 22(7): 648–54.

De Benedittis, G., and R. Massei. "Serotonin Precursors in Chronic Primary Headache: A Double-Blind Cross-Over Study with L-5-Hydroxytryptophan vs. Placebo." *Journal of Neurosurgical Sciences*, July–September 1985, 29(3): 239–48.

Meyers, S. "Use of Neurotransmitter Precursors for Treatment of Depression." *Alternative Medicine Review*, February 2000, 5(1): 64–71.

SAM-e

Bottiglieri, T., K. Hyland, and E. H. Reynolds. "The Clinical Potential of Ademetionine (S-Adenosylmethionine) in Neurological Disorders." *Drugs,* August 1994, 48(2): 137–52.

Bottiglieri, T., and K. Hyland. "S-Adenosylmethionine Levels in Psychiatric and Neurological Disorders: A Review." *Acta Neurologica Scandinavia Supplement,* 1994, 154: 19–26.

Bressa, G. M. "S-Adenosyl-L-Methionine (SAM-e) As Antidepressant: Meta-Analysis of Clinical Studies." *Acta Neurologica Scandinavia Supplement,* 1994, 154: 7–14.

Cantoni, G. L., S. H. Mudd, and V. Andreoli. "Affective Disorders and S-Adenosylmethionine: A New Hypothesis." *Trends in Neuroscience,* September 1989, 12(9): 319–24.

Rosenbaum, J. F., M. Fava, W. E. Falk, M. H. Pollack, L. S. Cohen, B. M. Cohen, and G. S. Zubenko. "The Antidepressant Potential of Oral S-Adenosyl-L-Methionine." *Acta Psychiatrica Scandinavia,* May 1990, 81(5): 432–36.

Salmaggi, P., G. M. Bressa, G. Nicchia, M. Coniglio, P. La Greca, and C. Le Grazie. "Double-Blind, Placebo-Controlled Study of S-Adenosyl-L-Methionine in Depressed Postmenopausal Women." *Psychotherapy and Psychosomatics,* 1993, 59(1): 34–40.

Resources

Numerous excellent resources are available on the topics of relaxation and other stress-management techniques, as well as exercise, diet, and supplements. A few of them are listed here.

Stress Management and Avoidance

Don't Sweat the Small Stuff—and It's All Small Stuff, by Richard Carlson (Hyperion, 1997)

Fight Fat after Forty, by Pamela Peeke (Penguin, 2001)

Simplify Your Life, by Elaine St. James (Hyperion, 1994)

Stress Management for Dummies, by Allen Elkin (For Dummies, 1999)

The Importance of Being Lazy, by Al Gini (Routledge, 2003)

Undoing Perpetual Stress, by Richard O'Connor (The Berkeley Publishing Group, 2005)

Why Zebras Don't Get Ulcers, by Robert M. Sapolsky (W. H. Freeman and Co., 1998)

You Can Choose to Be Happy, by Tom G. Stevens (Wheeler Sutton, 1998)

Exercise

Body for Life: Twelve Weeks to Mental and Physical Strength, by Bill Phillips and Michael D'Orso (HarperCollins, 1999)

The RealAge Workout, by Michael Roizen and Tracy Hafen (Collins, 2006)

The Strength and Toning Deck (cards), by Shirley Sugimura and Nicole Kaufman (Chronicle Books, 2004)

The Testosterone Advantage Plan: Lose Weight, Gain Muscle, Boost Energy, by Lou Schuler, Jeff Volek, Michael Mejia, and Andy Campbell (Fireside, 2002)

Weight-Walking: A New Path to Health and Fitness, by R. Schofield (Booksurge Publishing, 2006)

When Working Out Isn't Working Out, by Michael Gerrish (Griffin Trade Paperback, 1999)

Nutrition

Eat, Drink, and Be Healthy: The Harvard Medical School Guide to Healthy Eating, by Walter Willett, P. J. Skerrett, and Edward L. Giovannucci (Simon and Schuster, 2001)

Fad-Free Nutrition, by Frederick Stare and Elizabeth Whelan (Hunter House, 1998)

Mindless Eating: Why We Eat More than We Think, by Brian Wansink (Bantam, 2006)

Strong Women Eat Well: Nutritional Strategies for a Healthy Body and Mind, by Miriam E. Nelson and Judy Knipe (Putnam, 2001)

The Omnivore's Dilemma, by Michael Pollan (Penguin Press, 2006)

The Zone: Dietary Road Map to Losing Weight Permanently, by Barry Sears and Bill Lawren (HarperCollins, 1995)

What to Eat, by Marion Nestle (North Point Press, 2006)

Supplements

Chinese Herbal Medicine Made Easy: Effective and Natural Remedies for Common Illnesses, by Thomas Richard Joiner (Hunter House, 2001)

To find a qualified supplement consultant in your area, check with the following organizations:

American Nutraceutical Association: www.americanutra.com
American College of Nutrition: www.am-coll-nutr.org
American Dietetic Association: www.eatright.org
Other Books and Resources by Shawn M. Talbott

Cortisol Control and the Beauty Connection: The All-Natural, Inside-Out Approach to Reversing Wrinkles, Preventing Acne, and Improving Skin Tone, by Shawn M. Talbott (Hunter House, 2007)

The Cortisol Connection Diet: The Breakthrough Program to Control Stress and Lose Weight, by Shawn M. Talbott (Hunter House, 2004)

The Health Professional's Guide to Dietary Supplements, by Shawn M. Talbott and Kerry Hughes (Lippincott Williams and Wilkins, 2006)

Your Guide to Understanding Dietary Supplements: Magic Bullets or Modern Snake Oil? by Shawn M. Talbott (Haworth Press, 2003)

SupplementWatch website: www.SupplementWatch.com

Author's personal website: www.ShawnTalbott.com

Index